THE CARDIAC RECOVERY COOKBOOK

THE CARDIAC RECOVERY COOKBOOK

Heart-Healthy Recipes for Life After Heart Attack or Heart Surgery

M. Laurel Cutlip, R.D., L.N.

with **Sari Budgazad, R.D., C.D.N.**

Foreword by **Paul Kligfield, M.D.**

Medical Director, Cardiac Health Center
Weill-Cornell Center of The New-York Presbyterian Hospital

healthylivingbooks

New York • London

Library of Congress Cataloging-in-Publication Data

Cutlip, M. Laurel.
 The cardiac recovery cookbook : heart-healthy recipes for life after heart attack or heart surgery/
M. Laurel Cutlip with contributions by Sari Budgazad ; foreword by Paul Kligfield.
    p. cm.
ISBN 978-1-57826-189-5
1. Heart—Diseases—Diet therapy—Recipes. I. Budgazad, Sari. II. Title.
RC684.D5C88 2005
641.5'6311--dc22

                    2005001926

All Hatherleigh Press titles are available for bulk purchase, special promotions, and premiums. For more information, please contact the manager of our Special Sales Department at 1-800-528-2550.

Healthy Living Books
Hatherleigh Press
5-22 46th Avenue, Suite 200
Long Island City, NY 11101
1-800-528-2550

Interior designed by Deborah Miller and Eugenie Delaney
Cover Designed by Phil Mondestin and Deborah Miller

10 9 8 7 6 5

Portions of this book were previously published under the title *Keep the Beat: Heart-Healthy Recipes* from the National Heart, Lung, and Blood Institute. Hatherleigh Press assumes complete responsibility for this edition of the book.

Special thanks to Sari Budgazad, R.D., C.D.N., The New York-Presbyterian Hospital, Private Practice Nutrition Consultant. For an appointment, email sarird@aol.com.

Nutritional analyses of recipes on pages 21, 31, 32, 43, 45, 46, 54, 55, and 71 courtesy of Chef Kyle Shadix, R.D.C.C.C., M.S., R.D.

◆ ◆ ❖ ◆ ◆ ❖ ◆ ◆ ❖ ◆ ◆ ❖ ◆ ◆ ❖ ◆ ◆ ❖ ◆ ◆

U.S. Department of Health and Human Services
National Institutes of Health
National Heart, Lung, and Blood Institute

The recipes in this collection grew out of research and education projects supported by the National Heart, Lung, and Blood Institute. The studies and projects dealt with ways to help Americans keep their hearts strong by reducing their intake of calories, fat (especially saturated fat), cholesterol, and sodium. They include the Dietary Approaches to Stop Hypertension—or "DASH"—clinical study and the popular Stay Young at Heart nutrition education program. Now, you can use the results of these efforts to improve your heart health.

◆ ◆ ❖ ◆ ◆ ❖ ◆ ◆ ❖ ◆ ◆ ❖ ◆ ◆ ❖ ◆ ◆ ❖ ◆ ◆

Dedication

For my mentors, Kathie Morrison, Cathy and Don Wilson, and Kathy Marko.

For my friends, Jennifer and Kevin Ridgely, who have spent countless hours in hospital waiting rooms with me.

And for my family, who have the biggest and best hearts in the world.

Contents

◆ ◆ ❖ ◆ ◆ ❖ ◆ ◆ ❖ ◆ ◆ ❖ ◆ ◆ ◆ ◆ ❖ ◆ ◆ ❖ ◆ ◆

Foreword

◆ ◆ ❖ ◆ ◆ ❖ ◆ ◆ ❖ ◆ ◆ ❖ ◆ ◆ ❖ ◆ ◆ ❖ ◆ ◆

If you have picked up this book, chances are that you or someone you care about has had a heart attack, coronary artery bypass surgery, or angioplasty with a stent, or has been diagnosed with chronic disease of the coronary arteries or weakness of the heart muscle. Maybe you have already read *The Cardiac Recovery Handbook,* which focuses on medical management and lifestyle changes for patients with heart disease. You know that what someone eats can affect the course of the disease and recovery from disease. Diet is an important part of weight management and control of blood pressure. It is also critical to the limitation of atherosclerosis, which is the process that causes the arteries of the body to become clogged with fat and scar tissue. But sensible nutrition is not just a tool for recovery. When you think about it, it is pretty clear that what helps with recovery from heart disease should also be a useful way to prevent heart disease in the first place. So, this is a book that can benefit everyone.

This is not just another diet book or a book of favorite recipes. Remember, weight loss and protection of the heart can be distinct dietary goals. Because not all weight loss programs may confer the same benefit on the heart, it is essential that patients and their families understand the basic rationale of heart-healthy nutrition. *The Cardiac Recovery Cookbook* has grown out of the practical experience of two nutritionists who work with cardiac patients and their families on a daily basis. This experience is evident in the down-to-earth discussion of weight management. It is also obvious in the straightforward and understandable presentation of the basics of nutrition. You will learn about the different types of fats and oils and what makes them important for health. You will learn about the importance of vitamins and minerals in maintaining heart health. Tips on planning a nutritious day are well-organized and practically useful, and everyone should enjoy becoming a "savvy" supermarket shopper.

There was a time when nearly all heart-healthy diets were boring, and the rest were beyond boring. In describing the result of these diets, cynics used to say, wrongly: "It's not that you live longer, it just seems longer!" This is no longer the case. The many outstanding and delicious recipes presented in this book are not only heart-healthy, but they are fun to make and enjoyable to eat. Just take a look at the honey roasted almond crusted chicken with spinach and whole wheat couscous, as an example! You know that heart-healthy nutrition is the right thing to do, and it's time to get started. This book will help.

Paul Kligfield, M.D.
Medical Director, Cardiac Health Center
Weill-Cornell Center of
*   The New York-Presbyterian Hospital*

Preface

◆ ❖ ◆ ❖ ◆ ❖ ◆ ❖ ◆ ❖ ◆ ❖ ◆ ❖ ◆ ❖ ◆ ◆

It's hard to find anyone that hasn't in some way been affected by heart disease, the number one killer among Americans. People everywhere can be overheard giving nutritional advice—some accurate, some not so accurate. High blood pressure and cholesterol medications are heavily marketed in the media. Grocery stores are flooded with products geared to reducing dietary salt and fat and magazines offer "the diet of the week" to help fight the battle of the bulge.

Although I have been helping clients reduce their heart disease risk factors for nearly twenty years, it hit home about ten years ago when my father underwent cardiac bypass surgery as a result of having all four major heart arteries greater than 95 percent blocked. It was quite a shock. You see, Dad was an athlete and he never smoked. His weight was reasonable and he didn't have diabetes. He had high blood pressure and high cholesterol but they were under good control for years. He did, however, grow up in an Italian family consuming an enormous amount of cheese, sausage, salami, and ground beef. Although I tried to encourage both him and my mother to make dietary changes, they didn't listen—I guess that was retribution for my younger days of not listening to them (I, too, found out the hard way.) Dad also never had any symptoms. Yet, there he was on the gurney being prepared for major surgery.

Many people think of bypass surgery as low risk. Most people do fare well in the operating room, but many don't. Having been in the healthcare field for years, I was fully aware of that. Hours of waiting in the waiting room was both scary and stressful. You can't imagine how relieved I was to finally hear that all had gone well. Six years later, it was Mom's turn and things did not go so well. After five months of post-operative hospitalization, and complication after complication, we lost her. Then about two years ago, it struck again. My father-in-law underwent bypass surgery. Although I am glad to say that he is home, he had a rough time. His complication was a blood clot in his leg, amputated as a result.

You don't need to be the next in line. This book is more than just a cookbook, it is a facilitator of change! In addition to providing a wide assortment of great tasting recipes, you will learn the "whys" behind heart disease. We will cover common heart disease risk factors and discuss ways to eliminate as many of them as possible. Food labels will no longer be confusing and you will be able to use them with ease to quickly evaluate different products. Weight control tips, in addition to advice on how to alter favorite recipes, are provided. You will master ingredient selection and their proper storage. Distinguishing between the different types of fat, as well as fiber, and learning the food sources and desirable intakes of each, will be simple. Additionally, cooking methods to reduce sodium and fat are discussed in detail.

The time to change is NOW! I hope that each of you is motivated by the information we've provided, and as a result, lives a long, happy life. Good luck!

—M. Laurel Cutlip, R.D., L.N.

Abbreviations

Recipes use the following abbreviations:

lb	pound
oz	ounce
pt	pint
qt	quart
Tbsp	tablespoon
tsp	teaspoon

Nutrient lists use the following abbreviations:

g	gram
mg	milligram
%	percent

Chapter 1

◆ ◆ ❖ ◆ ◆ ❖ ◆ ◆ ❖ ◆ ◆ ❖ ◆ ◆ ❖ ◆ ◆ ❖ ◆ ◆

Introduction

Here's Some Terrific News!

Although heart disease is the number one killer among Americans, there are numerous paths you can take to prevent it from attacking you. Eating well is one of those avenues and heart-healthy eating really can taste great! Eating for the love of your heart doesn't mean turkey breast sandwiches for the rest of your life or an end to flavor or family favorites. It also doesn't mean that hours will be spent searching for special ingredients at the grocery store or slaving over the stove. The delicious, easily prepared recipes in this collection will lead the way and are sure to satisfy all of your family members, even the most finicky children. Watch their faces light up when they are served "Crispy Oven-Fried Chicken" with "Delicious Oven French Fries."

Variety is the spice of life and the recipes we've included, such as "Finger-Licking Curried Chicken," "Red Hot Fusilli" and "Beef Stroganoff" prove that cooking up heart health doesn't need to be boring. By altering a few simple ingredients to reduce sodium, saturated fat, cholesterol and calories, family favorites will be transformed into healthful dishes. The information that we provide will help you do just that—without sacrificing flavor.

Additionally, you will learn about heart disease risk factors and how the way you live your life impacts on them. Reading food labels with ease and utilizing them to make good choices will become second nature. Your awareness of the different types of fat and the benefits of fiber will increase. Furthermore, at the end of each recipe you will find a list of key nutrients to ensure that not only your heart, but also your entire body, is well nourished. BON APPETIT!

Eating for Heart Health—How Nutrition Affects Three Key Risk Factors

Feed your heart well and it will beat strong. Eat poorly and you are likely to develop three key factors that increase the risk of developing heart disease: high blood pressure, high blood cholesterol, and obesity.

Here's a brief look at why these three risk factors are so important:

Overweight and Obesity

More than fifty percent of Americans are overweight or obese. The resulting health complications are abundant. Not only does extra weight directly increase your risk of developing heart disease, it also makes you more likely to develop other conditions that increase heart disease risk. These factors include high blood pressure, high blood cholesterol and diabetes, all of which we will expand on later.

Achieving and maintaining a healthy weight is critical but unfortunately there is no magic wand available to help you reach this goal. However, understanding why weight gain occurs will help you make the proper adjustments. Just like our cars are powered by gas, our bodies are powered by calories. If you try to pump 21 gallons of gas in a 20-gallon gas tank, the gas will spill out all over your shoes. The same is true for your body. If you put more calories into your body then your body requires, you will spill out all over your jeans.

The amount of calories you consume through diet should not exceed the amount that you expend through body metabolism, such as breathing and digesting food, as well as that used during physical activity. If you eat more calories than needed, you'll gain weight.

Here's how to learn more about healthy eating as well as other heart health topics:
Write to the NHLBI Health Information Center
P.O. Box 30105
Bethesda, MD 20824-0105
Phone:(301) 592-8573
TTY: (240) 629-3255
Fax: (301) 592-8563
Visit the NHLBI online at: www.nhlbi.nih.gov at these special NHLBI Web pages:
For information about how to lose extra pounds or maintain a healthy weight:
www.nhlbi.nih.gov/health/public/heart/obesity/lose_wt
High blood pressure education can be found at:
www.nhlbi.nih.gov/hbp
To learn about high blood cholesterol visit: www.nhlbi.nih.gov/chd
Heart health for women information is found at: www.nhlbi.nih.gov/health/hearttruth

Even a modest decrease in calories consumed, however, can foster weight loss or, at a minimum, prevent you from gaining weight. If you are overweight, losing just ten percent of your current body weight helps to lower your risk of heart disease and improves your overall health significantly. If now is not an ideal time to put the effort into losing the extra weight, consider focusing on arresting further weight gain.

To determine if you are at an appropriate weight, use the following table called the body mass index (BMI). The BMI uses height and weight to determine body fat and applies to both adult men and women.

BMI CATEGORIES:
Underweight = <18.5
Normal weight = 18.5-24.9
Overweight = 25-29.9
Obesity = BMI of 30 or greater

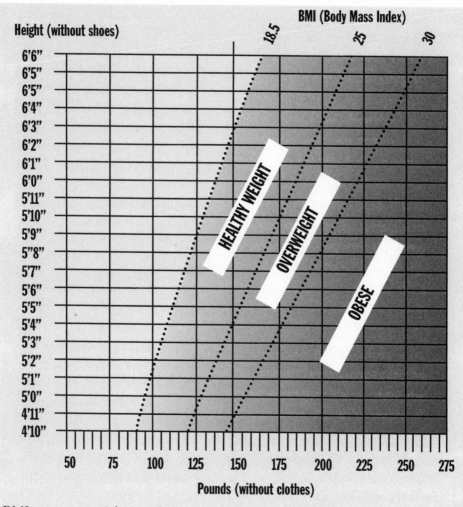

Pounds (without clothes)

BMI measures weight in relation to height. The BMI ranges shown above are for adults. They are not exact ranges of healthy and unhealthy weights. However, they show that health risk increases at higher levels of overweight and obesity. Even within the healthy BMI range, weight gains can carry health risks for adults.

Directions: Find your weight on the bottom of the graph. Go straight up from that point until you come to the line that matches your height. Then look to find your weight group.

Healthy Weight: BMI from 18.5 up to 25 refers to a healthy weight.
Overweight: BMI from 25 up to 30 refers to overweight.
Obese: BMI 30 or higher refers to obesity. Obese persons are also overweight.

If you are overweight, here are a few tips to help you keep your weight in check:

* *Pay attention to portion size. Large portions of even the healthiest of foods can lead to excessive calorie intake. Appropriate portion sizes will be discussed later.*

* *Choose fewer high-fat foods. High-fat foods often have more calories than other foods. Fat is like expensive high-octane gas; it costs nine calories per gram whereas protein and carbohydrate only cost four calories per gram.*

* *At the same time be wary of foods labeled "low-fat." Low-fat doesn't always mean low calorie. Extra sugars are often added to low-fat items, especially desserts, making them just as high in calories as regular versions of the same product.*

* *Choose foods with a high water content such as soups and fruits like oranges. Research has shown that foods containing a large amount of water tend to make you feel fuller. Foods with a high fiber content also foster satiety. These include whole grain breads and cereals, dry beans and peas, and fruits and vegetables.*

* *Be physically active. The more you move, the more calories your body needs. When you move your body, you not only burn calories, you build muscle. Muscle tissue requires significantly more calories than fat tissue does to maintain itself. Routine exercise has been linked to higher levels of good cholesterol (HDL), which protects the heart. Regular exercise also reduces the likelihood of developing high blood pressure, the risk factor we will discuss next.*

High Blood Pressure

Also called hypertension, high blood pressure is a condition that places you at risk for heart disease, stroke and kidney diseases. What is high blood pressure? High blood pressure is diagnosed when the force of blood against the walls of the arteries is too great, making your heart work harder than it should to pump blood throughout your body. About twenty-five percent of Americans have hypertension.

Diet plays an important role in your chance of developing high blood pressure. Controlling your weight by following an eating plan low in saturated fat and cholesterol and moderate in total fat is important for heart health generally and may help to prevent or control high blood pressure. Stress, alcohol, caffeine, low intakes of calcium, potassium, and magnesium, as well as certain dietary supplements and prescription drugs, may also influence blood pressure. A registered pharmacist can tell you if the drugs or supplements you take are altering your blood pressure.

Most people are aware that a high salt intake can adversely affect blood pressure. Since reducing dietary salt (sodium chloride) can prevent high blood pressure in those at risk, as well as help to control the disease in the older population, every effort should be made to reduce your intake of salt as well as other forms of sodium. Only small amounts of salt occur naturally in foods. Most of the salt consumed by Americans is added during food processing, in food preparation at home, or in a restaurant. The American Heart Association recommends that you consume no more than 6 grams (about 1 teaspoon) of table salt a day. That equals 2.4 grams (2,400 milligrams) of sodium a day. By further reducing table salt to 4 grams (or 2/3 teaspoon) a day, studies such as the Dietary Approaches to Stop Hypertension trial (DASH) indicate that many people are able to control or prevent the condition. Four grams of salt is equal to 1.5 grams (1,500 milligrams) of sodium a day. The above recommendations include ALL salt and sodium consumed—that added during cooking, at the table, as well as what is present in prepared and processed foods. After about two months of cutting back on salt, most people lose their craving for it.

High Blood Cholesterol

Fat and cholesterol in the diet can raise the level of cholesterol in the blood, and that can lead to atherosclerosis, a type of hardening of the arteries. In atherosclerosis, cholesterol, fat, and other substances build up in the inner portions of artery walls. As the process continues, arteries, including those to the heart, may narrow, reducing blood flow. Saturated fat is a type of fat that is generally solid at room temperature. This fat causes blood cholesterol to rise more than anything else in the diet. Some examples of foods high in saturated fat include: meat, cheese, butter and many processed foods. By choosing low-fat or fat-free items, especially in the dairy case, you can reduce your saturated fat intake immensely—but, again, keep an eye on the products' calorie content. Too much of a good thing can lead to weight gain.

Some foods can actually help to lower blood cholesterol. Foods containing soluble (also called viscous) fiber are one such category. Soluble fiber is found in cereal grains, fruits, vegetables, and legumes (like dried beans, peas, and lentils). We will discuss fiber more completely a little later.

Other food products that lower blood cholesterol are those containing plant stanols or plant sterols. When consumed, these extracts found in some plants including soy and pine needles, inhibit the absorption of cholesterol in the small intestine. Cholesterol-lowering spreads such as "Benechol" and "Take Control" fall into this category. Plant stanols and sterols are noted on the products food label.

Reduce Your Heart Disease Risk

Anyone could be a victim of heart disease. Contrary to popular belief, heart disease strikes women as often as it does men. Each of us has the ability to reduce our chance of developing the disease by preventing or controlling behaviors and conditions known to increase its risk. They're called "risk factors," and there are two types: those you can't change and those you can. Uncontrollable risk factors that you can't alter are your age (45 or older for men, 55 or older for women) and having a family history of early heart disease (a father or brother diagnosed before age 55, or a mother or sister diagnosed before age 65). Controllable risk factors include: smoking, high blood pressure, high blood cholesterol, overweight/ obesity, physical inactivity, and diabetes. Now let's talk a little about each of these.

If you smoke, stop. Smoking more than doubles your risk of having a heart attack and if you do have one, you are more likely to die. It has also been linked to lower levels of HDL, the protective blood cholesterol. If you haven't been able to quit in the past, keep trying. Consider asking your doctor about local smoking cessation programs or for medication that may help reduce your desire to smoke.

Control high blood pressure. There are few warning signs for high blood pressure, so have your blood pressure checked regularly (once every 2 years if it is normal, more often if it is not). Also, maintain a healthy weight and limit your intake of alcoholic beverages to one drink per day for women and two for men.

Reduce high blood cholesterol. Maintain a healthy weight and get your cholesterol level checked once every 5 years (more often, if it's been high in the past). This test measures the level of cholesterol circulating in the bloodstream. Aim for a total cholesterol below 200, a good cholesterol "HDL" above 40 and a bad "LDL" cholesterol under 100.

Keep your weight in check. Carrying extra weight puts a big strain on your heart. To lose weight and keep it off, adopt a lifestyle that combines sensible eating with regular physical activity. If past attempts at weight loss have ended in failure, consider getting help from a qualified health professional such as a registered dietitian, who can tailor a nutrition plan to your specific needs.

Increase your activity level. Try to engage in at least 30 minutes of moderate-intensity physical activity, such as brisk walking, on most and preferably all days of the week. The 2005 USDA Dietary Guidelines increased this recommendation to 60 minutes, but even increasing your activity level by a small amount can help reduce your heart disease risk. Take the stairs, hide the TV remote, or get on and off your commuter train or bus a stop early and walk the rest of the way.

Prevent or control diabetes. Many of the steps that lower your risk of heart disease also reduce your chance of developing diabetes. If you already have diabetes check your blood sugar frequently to make sure it falls within a desirable range. New medications and flexible eating plans make controlling blood sugar much easier than it has previously been. Ask your physician for guidance and attend diabetic classes. Also be sure to routinely monitor your blood sugar; uncontrolled diabetes significantly damages the heart.

Chapter 2

◆ ◆ ❖ ◆ ◆ ◆ ❖ ◆ ◆ ◆ ❖ ◆ ◆ ◆ ❖ ◆ ◆ ◆ ❖ ◆ ◆

Weight Management and Dieting

Weight Management

Weight management is an important component of adapting a heart-healthy lifestyle. The Body Mass Index (BMI) chart provided is one tool that can be used to identify your weight category. If your BMI is greater than 25, you may benefit from losing weight. If you are at a normal weight, it is still a good idea to learn your daily calorie needs and use them as a base for making nutritious food choices. Many of the heart disease risk factors described earlier tend to occur together and, to some extent, are influenced by your eating habits. If you have at least three of the following—high triglycerides, high blood pressure, low HDL, and abdominal obesity—you have what is now called metabolic syndrome. For this reason, a well-balanced diet that fits your individual calorie needs should be the first line of defense against cardiovascular disease.

The Dangers of Dieting

In order to simplify the advice on slimming down, let's first dispel common diet myths. Many popular diets promise instant weight reduction, but they are lacking in heart-healthy nutrients. Furthermore, diets that promote one food or eliminating entire food groups are difficult to follow for long periods of time. It is unrealistic to expect one to eat grapefruit, cabbage soup, or peanut butter every single day without getting bored! On the other hand, Weight Watchers is a helpful weight loss tool because it promotes sensible eating without reducing dietary variety. With that said, here are a few tips to help you spot a diet with misleading claims:

* *If a diet sounds too good to be true, it probably is. Products and programs that promise quick and "magic" results are misleading since successful weight loss is a gradual process that requires lifestyle changes.*

* *Any ad that recommends more than 1 to 2 pounds of weight loss per week is not safe.*

* *Diets that have a list of forbidden foods should be avoided. Depriving yourself of your favorite foods may lead to future binges.*

* *Keep your eye out for diets that require special food or supplements. "Natural" or "herbal" supplements are not regulated by the Food and Drug Administration, and allow manufacturers to market practically anything as a diet aid. This is a major health concern in light of Fen/Phen and Ephedrine related deaths over the past few years. Red flag: these products are often promoted using anecdotal reports instead of reliable scientific evidence.*

* *If the diet does not mention the importance of exercise, don't buy into it. Once you learn how to eat nutritiously, exercise is what really helps keep the weight off. Aerobic exercises such as swimming or jogging are fat-burning activities. Resistance training such as exercising with free weights will help build muscle mass. Exercise is a built-in security tool to eating healthy. For example, you might think twice about eating a piece of cake if you know it requires 45 minutes on the treadmill to burn it off!*

In addition, let's address the specific dangers of some popular diets. Meal replacement diets, for instance, do not work in the long term. While you may initially lose weight due to drastically reducing your calorie intake, the problem arises when you go off the diet. Face it, you are not going to drink shakes for the rest of your life. The diet is a temporary solution to shedding a few pounds, but it fails to teach one how to plan balanced, nutritious meals.

What about high protein, low-carbohydrate diets? These diets promote a very low-carbohydrate intake, 30 grams or less a day. We store carbohydrates in the form of glycogen. As you lower your carbohydrate intake, your body uses glycogen stores for energy. The glycogen that is released is bound to three water molecules. Thus, initial weight loss is a result of fluid loss and dehydration. Loss of water weight is often mistaken for "fat loss." When the body is void of carbohydrates as an energy source, it burns fat for energy in the form of ketones. Ketosis can create an imbalance of electrolytes in your body (which can lead to heart failiure), cause calcium to be leached from the bones, and burden your kidneys.

Low-carbohydrate diets have also been associated with decreased concentration (since carbohydrate is the brain's primary fuel source), headaches, nausea, bad breath, and hair loss. In addition, scientific studies have not confirmed long-term health benefits of following a low-carbohydrate diet. Let's not neglect to mention that high protein diets allow unlimited quantities of foods high in artery-clogging saturated fats such as bacon, steak, and cheese.

If you decide to restrict high quality carbohydrates from your diet, there is a price to pay. By banning a baked potato with skin, you miss out on vitamin C and fiber. If you favor a processed protein bar over a fresh fruit salad, you lose out on the naturally occurring nutrients and phytochemicals that whole foods contain. It becomes more difficult to meet your B vitamin needs without eating whole grain cereals and breads. Furthermore, these diets require you to take nutrient supplements, which can burn a hole in your wallet. The vitamins, minerals and antioxidants found in whole fruits and vegetables are cheaper and serve as natural protectors against chronic diseases.

Diets that are below 1000 calories can also be dangerous. While it is true that weight loss is achieved by combining a reduced calorie intake with regular physical activity, very low calorie diets are nutritionally inadequate and can slow down your metabolism. Still not convinced? A major calorie deficit puts your body on the defense. Imagine that you are stranded in the middle of the Sahara desert without food or water. Your body is naturally designed to burn calories less efficiently in order to preserve fat and muscle mass. Similarly, when you eat too little, it is even more difficult to lose weight in the long run!

Weight loss that works against health gains is a dangerous result of fad dieting. Rather than plugging yourself into someone else's diet system, use your personal eating habits and favorite foods as a base for healthy modification. The following guidelines will teach you how to calculate your calorie needs and design a personal eating pattern using the exchange lists for weight management. Remember there are no good or bad foods as long as you keep portions under control, while still enjoying the taste of nature's finest foods.

How to Use the Exchange Lists

The exchange lists are foods grouped together because of their similar nutritional content. Each serving of a food has about the same amount of carbohydrates, fat, protein, and calories as the other foods on that list. For example, you can trade a slice of low-fat cheese for a slice of Healthy choice turkey meat. Each of these foods equals one lean protein choice. Another example is trading a small baked potato for a ½ cup pasta. Each of these foods equals one starch choice.

How many servings do you need from each exchange group?

Once you calculate your calorie needs, the sample diet plans provided will tell you how many servings from each food group to eat. Please note that the low glycemic index eating plan is not a low-carbohydrate diet. This diet plan limits refined carbohydrates (white rice, white bread, muffins, cookies, potato chips, etc), and promotes a sensible intake of low calorie, high-fiber carbohydrates to support heart health.

How many calories should you consume each day?

Step 1: Personalize your Calorie Needs

If you are sedentary or lightly active throughout the day, multiply your body weight by 13.

If you are moderately active, (30 to 45 minutes of walking, biking, aerobic activity 3 times per week), multiply your body weight by 15.

Step 2: Fat Calories

Your fat intake should be controlled but not eliminated from your diet. A heart-healthy recommendation is to consume less than 30% of calories from fat.

Step 3: To Lose Weight

Research suggests that losing ½ to 1 pound a week by eating better and exercising more is the best way to lose weight and keep it off! You would need to consume 3500 extra calories to gain one pound. To lose weight sensibly, subtract 500 calories a day from your total daily calorie requirement.

Example:

Ms. Smith weighs 150 pounds. She spends most of her day at the office and one hour doing chores around the house.

Estimate daily calorie requirement: 150 x 13 = 1950 calories / day

Estimate daily fat requirement: 1950 x 0.3 (30%) = 585 fat calories / day

To lose weight, Ms. Smith would decrease her calorie intake to 1950-500 = 1450 calories / day

To boost her metabolism, she can also increase her daily physical activity.

Remember:

Very low calorie diets (less than 1000 calories per day) are dangerous, preventing you from getting all the nutrients you need. Eating too few calories can slow your body's metabolism.

Tips to help you get started:

* *Combine at least 3 food groups at meals. For example, scoop out a bagel to decrease the calorie content from the dough (enriched flour) and spread 1 teaspoon of peanut with sliced bananas for a more balanced meal that contains unsaturated fat, protein, potassium, and B vitamins.*

* *Pay close attention to how much you eat. The reason why only 7% of the population in France is obese compared to 30% of Americans has little to do with genetics or drinking red wine. Preventing weight gain is due to eating moderately sized portions from each food group.*

* *Eat slowly! It takes 20 minutes for the brain to register that you feel full from a meal. It is very easy to exceed your calorie limit in that time period if you eat rapidly.*

Sample Diet Plans

Low-fat diet (approximately 55 to 60% carbohydrate, 20% fats, 20 to 25% protein). The diet plan recommended for most people is one that is low-fat, and moderate in carbohydrates and protein.

	1200 calories	1500 calories	1800 calories
Lean protein (per oz)	6	7	8
Starches	5	7	8
Vegetables	4+	4+	4+
Fruits	3	4	5
Fats	1	2	3
Dairy (nonfat or 1%)*	2	2	2

Low glycemic index diet (approximately 45 to 50% carbohydrates, 25 to 30% protein and 25 to 30% fats) is indicated for those people who have difficulty losing weight on the typical low-fat diet. This diet emphasizes fibrous vegetables and legumes rather than simple carbohydrates and starches made from refined starches. It is slightly higher in protein and fat. Try to select unsaturated sources of fat such as olive oil and nuts versus saturated fats such as butter.

	1200 calories	1500 calories	1800 calories
Lean protein (per oz)	7	8	9
Starches	3	4	5
Vegetables	7+	7+	7+
Fruits	2	3	4
Fats	2	4	5
Dairy (nonfat or 1%)*	2	2	2

* Depending on the dairy sources consumed, a calcium supplement may be necessary for 100% of the requirements to be met.

Exchange List for Weight Management: Heart-Healthy Choices

BREAD/STARCH

Choose 3-8 servings daily
1 serving =
15 grams carbohydrates
3 grams protein
80 calories

dry cereal
unsweetened	¾ cup
cooked cereal	½ cup

bread 1 slice
bun (hamburger)	½
bun (hot dog)	½
bagel (Lenders)	½

dried beans
cooked	⅓ cup
baked	¼ cup
corn	½ cup
lima beans	½ cup
potato (baked)	small
potato (mashed)	½ cup
winter squash	1 cup
popcorn	3 cups

(popped without fat)
pretzels	¾ oz
pasta (cooked)	½ cup
brown rice	⅓ cup
yam sweet potato	½ cup

VEGETABLES

Choose 4+ servings daily
½ cup cooked or 1 cup raw
7 grams carbohydrates
2 grams protein
25 calories

arugula
asparagus
beans (green wax)
beets
broccoli
brussel sprouts
cabbage
carrots
cauliflower
celery
cucumber
green pepper
mushrooms (cooked)
okra
onions
spinach
tomatoes
turnips

FRUIT:

Choose 2-5 servings daily
1 serving =
15 grams carbohydrates
60 calories

apple	1 small
apricot	½ cup
banana	½
cantaloupe (cubed)	1 cup
cherries	½ cup
grapefruit	½ medium
grapes	½ cup (17)
orange	1 medium
peach	1 medium
pear	1 medium
pineapple	¾ cup
raspberries	1 cup
strawberries	1¼ cup
watermelon	1¼ cup cubes
fruit juices	⅓–½ cup
dried fruit	¼ cup

MEAT AND SUBSTITUTES

Choose 5-9 ounces daily
1 oz serving =
7 grams protein
1-3 grams fat
35-55 calories

beef, lean only
round steak	1 oz
flank steak	1 oz
tenderloin, pork	1 oz
tenderloin, ham	1 oz
Canadian bacon	1 oz
Veal	1 oz

poultry (no skin)
chicken	1 oz
turkey	1 oz

fish
fresh/frozen	1 oz
canned in water	2 oz
	(¼ c)
shellfish	2 oz
cottage cheese	¼ cup
parmesan (grated)	2 Tbsp
low-fat	1 oz

(less than 55 calories per ounce)

peanut butter ,	1 Tbsp
(all natural)	
lunch meat (95% fat-free)	1 slice
tofu	½ cup
egg whites	2
egg substitutes	¼ cup

* Note: 3oz serving of meat =
deck of cards/ palm of hand

MILK:

Choose 2 servings daily
1 serving =
12 grams carbohydrates
8 grams protein
1-2 grams fat
90-120 calories

milk (skim/skim plus),	1 cup
soy milk (low-fat),	1 cup
yogurt (nonfat/lite),	1 cup
hot chocolate (lite),	1 cup
pudding	½ cup
(fat-free/sugar-free)	

FAT

Choose only 2-4 servings
1 serving =
1 tsp regular or 1 Tbsp lite
5 grams fat
45 calories

UNSATURATED
avocado	⅛ medium
margarine	1 tsp
mayonnaise	1 tsp
cashews, almonds	6
pecans	4 halves
peanuts	10
olives	5
salad dressing	1 Tbsp
oils	1 tsp

corn
cottonseed
safflower
soybean
sunflower
olive
peanut
canola
tahini paste	2 tsp
peanut butter	2 tsp

Spotlight on the South Beach Diet

From bunless burgers to protein bars, the low–carbohydrate (carb) craze is being embraced by fast food chains and supermarkets nationwide. So, are you wondering if eating low-carb foods will help you lose weight?

The Claims: Excess weight comes from highly processed carbs that we eat found in baked goods, breads, and snacks. Cutting bad carbs can help decrease hunger, reduce insulin resistance, promote weight loss, and improve blood lipids.

The South Beach Diet is divided into three phases. Phase one lasts two weeks, and no carbohydrates are allowed to be eaten (grains, milk, fruits, vegetables). By week three, you can add some bread, fruit, and carb-containing snacks to your diet, resulting in further weight loss (1 to 2 pounds/week). Phase three allows you to resume a regular diet with an emphasis on unrefined carbs. The diet claims you will still lose weight because you lose your urge to eat refined carbs.

Although it allows ample fat and protein, the author does promotes foods lower in saturated fat, sodium, and cholesterol (such as lean beef, pork, and veal, olive/canola oil, low-fat dairy, and nuts). In addition, he distinguishes wholesome carbohydrates (fiber-rich fruits, vegetables, and whole grains) from refined carbohydrates.

Rapid weight loss during phase one is most likely due to loss of water weight. South Beach is basically a "modified Atkins." There is also no mention of physical activity, a valuable component in sustaining weight loss. While the diet may be helpful for people with insulin resistance, it is not as applicable to a healthy individual just trying to lose a few pounds. There is also lack of research to support long-term benefits of eating the South Beach way. It fails to teach one *how* to adapt healthful eating behaviors. Instead, it fosters erratic eating patterns. The book recommends that if you overindulge in carbs during phase two, resume phase one until you lose the desired weight. Reality check . . . it's excess calorie intake, not carb intake, that is the culprit for weight gain!

Low-Carb does not equal Low Calorie

Low-Carb Option:

Sandwich #1
2 slices of low-carb Atkins bread:
129 calories
1 slice low-fat cheese:
55 calories
1 oz low-carb chocolate bar:
155 calories
Total: 339 calories

Snack #1
3 low-carb Entenmanns
cookies: 130 calories
1 cup of 2% milk: 120 calories
Total: 250 calories

Balanced Meal:

Sandwich #2
2 slices of reduced-calorie whole
wheat bread: 100 calories 1 slice
of low-fat alpine lace cheese:
55 calories
1 oz Healthy Choice turkey/1.5 oz
tuna in water: 55 calories
1 cup chopped: spinach, tomato,
scallions, carrots, peppers,
cucumbers 25 calories
½ cup cherries and blueberries,
or fresh peach or pear: 60 calories
Total: 295 calories

Snack #2
1 Tbsp peanut butter and
4 honey-wheat pretzels : 155
1 cup of fat-free milk: 90 calories
Total: 245 calories

The bottom line is low-carb foods are not more nutritious or less caloric than most regular foods, and are usually more expensive than healthy natural foods.

The Dietitian's Advice

There is little evidence for the claim that some types of carbs are more likely to cause weight gain than others just because they affect blood sugar faster. Insulin is a hormone that is needed for the transfer of sugar, along with protein and fat out of the blood and into the cells for energy. It is often mistakenly considered a "fat storage hormone." While it is true that carbohydrate containing foods turn to sugar and drive up insulin levels, the majority of people do not secrete excess insulin in response to eating

The Low-Carb Lingo

While the changes manufacturers take to reduce the carbs in various foods are not necessarily unhealthy, the amount of calories themselves are not changed. Low-carb products end up having nearly as many calories as their regular counterparts.

Refined wheat flour is frequently replaced with soy flour (higher in protein), soy protein, or wheat protein. Extra fiber, such as wheat bran, oat bran, or other fiber is added with additional high-fat ingredients. Manufacturers also replace sugar with sugar alcohols (maltitol, lactitol, or sorbitol) or artificial sweeteners. This is the same stuff found in sugarless candies.

In low-carb beers, they use chemicals in the brewing process to reduce the carbs in the brew, but the result in not very different from common "lite" beers in the market. For example, a 12 ounce can of Michelob Ultra "low-carb" has 95 calories, and 2.6 grams of carbs. Coors lite has 102 calories and 5 grams of carbs, a very tiny difference!

If you are attracted to these new products, keep in mind that the FDA has not yet approved low-carb labeling. If you are trying to manage your weight, cutting calories and increasing physical activity is the key. Protein has as many calories as carbs do, and fat has more than twice as many calories. According to food label law, bread must have less than 3 grams of fat per serving to be called low-fat, but any bread can be called low-carb.

Net carbs are translated as the carbohydrates in a food that affect blood sugar. Fiber and sugar alcohols do not count. So if a food has 10 grams of carbs, but 6 grams are fiber, the product is advertised as 4 "net impact" carbs.

moderatelysized portions of carbohydrates. There are many factors that regulate hunger and satiety aside from the glycemic index of foods, (a rating scale of how quickly food is turned into glucose). Focus more on the nutritional quality of your entire meal—eating sensible portions of wholesome carbs, lean sources of protein, and unsaturated fats.

Planning your Plate Using Carb Counting

Counting carbohydrates may be useful if you have diabetes or insulin resistance. The following meal ideas will guide you in incorporating sensible portions of wholesome carbohydrates at each meal. Remember to choose foods that offer the most nutrients per serving. If the bulk of your diet consists of whole grains, lean sources of protein, low-fat dairy foods, unsaturated fats, fruits and vegetables, then a piece of cake or a glass of wine won't tip the scale!

1 Carb choice = 15 grams

BREAKFAST TIME:
Choose a protein or high-fiber starch base for the meal.

Example of a starch base:
- Whole wheat pita loaf, 2 tsp of peanut butter, ½ banana, sliced
  TOTAL: 300 calories, 3 carbs
- Bakery Bagel TOTAL: 400 calories, 5 carbs (75 grams)

Example of a protein base:
- Egg whites with low-fat shredded cheese, ½ cup chopped veggies, Dole fruit cup TOTAL: 250 calories, 2 carbs (30 grams)

SNACK TIME:
Choose a high fiber snack such as fruits and vegetables.
- ¼ cup dried fruit, 1 small fruit TOTAL: 1 carb choice

Other snack ideas that count as 1 carb choice:

3 graham cracker squares	½ cup unsweetened applesauce
2 rice cakes	1 cup fruit flavored yogurt sweetened
15 to 20 fat-free snack chips	with sugar substitute
2 to 4 whole wheat crackers	½ cup sugar-free pudding
1 cup mixed vegetables with corn, peas, or pasta	⅓ cup low-fat frozen yogurt
3 cups popped fat-free popcorn	1 cup melon cubes

Mix these carb choices with protein/healthy fats:
Vegetables with 1 Tbsp hummus
1 cup melon cubes with ¼ cup low-fat cottage cheese
2 to 4 crackers with 2 tsp of all-natural peanut butter
1 cup plain yogurt topped 1 handful of almonds, soy nuts,
   trail mix of ¼ cup dried fruit with nuts

LUNCH TIME:
Choose a soup/salad/sandwich base
Soups:
(1 cup=1 carb choice)
    bean   chicken noodle
    vegetable   tomato made with water

(½ cup=1 carb choice)
split pea

Salad: with vinegar/oil dressing
Romaine
green leaf lettuce
spinach (add 2 to 3 ounces protein)

Adding carbs to a salad bar meal:
1 carb choice
    1 small roll   corn   1 small potato
    ½ cup beans   ½ cup pasta

Sandwich:
(1 carb choice=1 slice)
    100% whole wheat bread
    rye
    pumpernickel

Veggie Sandwich:
avocado slices   onion
alfalfa sprouts   cucumber
shredded carrots   cherry tomatoes
Add: ¼ cup tuna/salmon (canned in water, prepared with fat-free mayonnaise)

Pizza:
Pros: Pizza provides a variety of nutrients such as protein calcium, fiber (whole grain crust). **Cons:** Calories add up fast, and are high in saturated fat so keep the portions sensible. Eat 1 slice with a side salad/or vegetable topping on pizza
Sbarro's cheese pizza: 4 carb choices (60 grams), 455 calories, 13 grams fat
Papa John's: (⅛ of whole 14" pizza): Garden special: 2.5 carb choices (38 grams) 280 calories, 10 grams fat
Domino's: 2 slices of medium thin crust pizza: 2 carb choices (31 grams) 275 calories, 12 grams fat

SNACK TIME:
Refer to snack ideas outlined above.

DINNER TIME:
Stir fry vegetables in 2 teaspoons olive oil
Eat over 1 cup pasta, ⅔ cup of rice (2 carb choices) or wrap vegetables in a whole wheat tortilla (1 6" tortilla=carb choice)
Add protein: steamed shrimp, tofu, grilled chicken

Sample Recipe:
Honey Roasted Almond Chicken with Spinach and Whole Wheat Couscous

1   12-oz box of whole wheat couscous
4   4-oz boneless, skinless chicken breasts (fat trimmed off)
    garlic powder to taste
    pepper to taste
2   Tbsp all purpose flour
¼   cup egg beaters or 2 egg whites
½   cup honey roasted almond slivers
1   Tbsp olive oil
1   lb bag of fresh spinach (yields 1½ cups cooked)
1   Tbsp chopped garlic (optional)
1   Tbsp lemon juice (optional)

NUTRITIONAL FACTS	
CALORIES:	560.40KCALS
PROTEIN:	44.17G
CARBS:	64.94G
TOTAL FAT:	15.40G
SAT FAT:	1.73G
CHOLESTEROL:	65.77MG
SODIUM:	392.95MG
FIBER:	13.48G
CALCIUM:	198.21MG
POTASSIUM:	841.30MG
YIELD:	4 SERVINGS
EXCHANGES PER SERVING:	
4 STARCHES, 4 LEAN PROTEIN, 1 FAT	
SERVING SIZE: 1 (4 OZ) CHICKEN BREAST WITH ⅛ CUP ALMONDS, ½ CUP OF COUSCOUS, ½ CUP SPINACH	

1. Prepare couscous according to package directions.
2. Season chicken breasts with pepper and garlic powder. Coat both sides in flour.
3. Dip flour-coated chicken breasts in egg beaters.
4. Press almonds into both sides of chicken breast.
5. Heat oil in skillet and cook chicken breast on each side over medium-high heat until no longer pink.
6. To steam spinach: wash thoroughly, tear off stems. Place the spinach in a microwave safe dish and add ½ inch of water. Cover with lid and microwave on high for 4 minutes. Toss with a little lemon juice if desired. Another good addition is chopped garlic.
7. Serve chicken breast on bed of spinach with couscous on the side.

This recipe is full of flavor without the use of salt or high sodium marinades. It offers a nice balance of high-fiber starch, lean protein, and unsaturated fats (olive oil).

Chapter 3

❖ ◆ ❖ ◆ ❖ ◆ ❖ ◆ ❖ ◆ ❖ ◆ ❖ ◆ ❖ ◆ ❖ ◆ ❖

Spotlight on Vegetarian Diets

Vegetarian is a basic term used to describe people who exclude meat, milk, poultry, fish or other animal derived foods from their diet. Lacto-ovo-vegetarian is the most liberal type, and refers to people who eat dairy products and eggs, but exclude meat, fish, poultry, and seafood. Vegan refers to strict vegetarians who exclude all animal derived foods such as meat, poultry, fish, seafood, eggs, and dairy products.

The dietary factor most directly related to coronary artery disease is saturated animal fat. Fewer vegetarians than meat eaters suffer from diseases of the heart and arteries because their diets are generally lower in saturated fat and cholesterol. In addition, plant-based diets tend to be higher in heart-healthy fats such as seeds, nuts, and vegetable oils. Furthermore, studies have shown that people who eat a healthy vegetarian diet have lower rates of hyperlipidemia (high levels of blood fats), hypertension, cancer, obesity, and diabetes.

If not properly balanced, a vegetarian diet can lack essential nutrients such as protein, iron, calcium, vitamin D, vitamin B12, and zinc. Lacto-ovo-vegetarians who use animal derived foods such as milk and eggs receive high quality protein and are unlikely to develop deficiencies. Vegans can meet their protein needs by eating a wide variety of complementary foods including whole grains, legumes, seeds, nuts, textured vegetable protein (soy protein), and vegetables. If you are a vegetarian or just interested in substituting animal derived foods for plant based foods, use the following guidelines to meet your nutritional needs.

Nutrients of concern when planning a vegetarian diet

Iron. Iron is an essential mineral that carries oxygen to cells to make energy (iron is a component of body proteins such as hemoglobin and myoglobin). Iron also helps keep your immune system operating at peak efficiency. Vegetarian food sources include lentils, chickpeas, swiss chard, tofu, pumpkin seeds, and enriched cereals.

> Recommended Dietary Allowance (RDA):
> Males: 9–13 years: 8 mg/day
> Males: 11–50 years: 11 mg/day
> Males: 19+ years: 8 mg/day
>
> Females: 9–13 years: 8 mg/day
> Females: 14–18 years: 15 mg/day
> Females: 19–50 years: 18 mg/day
> Females: 51+ years: 8 mg/day

Calcium. Calcium is an essential mineral that helps build strong bones. Calcium also helps muscles contract, helps blood clot, and plays a role in normal nerve function. Vegetarian food sources include non-fat yogurt, milk, low-fat cheese, fortified soymilk/orange juice, tofu made with calcium sulfate, kale, broccoli, and bok choy. Spinach, rhubarb, and swiss chard contain calcium, but are not as absorbable.

> RDA:
> Males and Females 19-50 yrs: 1000 mg/day
> Males and Females 51+ yrs: 1200 mg/day

Vitamin D. Vitamin D promotes absorption of minerals in the body (calcium and phosphorous) and helps deposit them in the bones and teeth. Vegetarian food sources include fortified milk/soymilk, low-fat cheese, eggs/egg scramblers, fortified cereals, and soft non-hydrogenated margarines (read the label to make sure that the margarine is made with canola or olive oil). A natural source of vitamin D is exposure to sunlight!

Adequate intake (AI):
Males and Females 25-50 yrs: 5 mcg/day (200 IU)
Males and females 51-70 years: 10 mcg/day (400 IU)
Males and females 70+ years: 15 mcg/day (600 IU)

Vitamin B12. Vitamin B12 works with folate to make red blood cells. Vitamin B12 also serves as a vital part of many body chemicals, helping the body use fatty acids and amino acids. Vegetarian food sources include fortified cereals, soy beverages, and some brands of nutritional yeast. Tempeh (a cultured soy food with a mushroom like flavor), seaweed, spirulina, and other fermented foods are unreliable sources. Vitamin B12 supplements (in the form of cyanocobalamin) may be recommended for vegetarians over 50 years who do not eat these specified food items.

RDA:
Males and Females 14-70 yrs: 2.4 mcg/day

Zinc. Zinc is an essential mineral for growth. Zinc promotes cell production, tissue growth and repair, and wound healing. It is required for energy metabolism and helps utilize carbohydrate, protein, and fat. Vegetarian food sources include whole grain products, wheat bran, soybeans, and legumes.

RDA:
Males: 11+ years: 15 mg/day
Females 11+: 12 mg/day

Are you a meat eater or plant eater? Omnivores refer to people who have no formal restriction on the eating of any foods. An omnivore does not have to become a strict vegetarian to reap the benefits of a plant-based diet. In fact, adapting a vegetarian diet can help you meet heart-healthy nutrition guidelines. Simply increasing your intake of fruits, vegetables, whole grains, legumes, and tofu offers significant health advantages. Keep in mind that both plant-based and meat-based diets can become unhealthy when overloaded with fat and empty calories. The following example highlights the importance of nutritious meal planning:

What's wrong with the following lacto-ovo-vegetarian lunch?

Appetizer: corn chips with sour cream
Entrée: grilled cheese prepared in butter with french fries, 1 cup whole milk OR
fried egg on a roll with hash browns, 1 cup whole milk
Dessert: ice cream with Reeses Peanut Butter pieces

Healthier lacto-ovo-vegetarian lunch:

Appetizer: fresh broccoli, carrots with low-fat vegetable dip
Entrée: vegetable quesadilla prepared with soy cheese on a whole wheat tortilla OR
vegetarian chile (beans, onions, peppers, garlic, low sodium tomatoes, bulgur, spices) with 1 cup fortified soymilk/skim milk
Dessert: fresh fruit salad OR low-fat frozen yogurt topped with soy nuts

Remember that the foods you exclude are not nearly important as the foods you include in your diet. Planning healthy vegetarian meals involves incorporating foods low in saturated fat, cholesterol, and sodium, but high in antioxidants (vitamin A, vitamin C), folate, and fiber. A vegetarian diet can meet all your nutritional needs, as long as you increase diet variety!

A Guide to Buying and Using Tofu

Tofu is made by a process similar to cheese making. The soybeans are soaked, ground with water, and cooked. The soymilk is filtered out from the solids and coagulated. Tofu is an excellent source of soy protein. The Food and Drug Administration allows foods that contain at least 6.25 grams of soy protein per serving to carry this health claim on the package: *"Diets low in saturated fat and cholesterol that include 25 grams of soy protein a day may reduce the risk of heart disease."* The foods must also meet the criteria for low-fat, low saturated fat, and low cholesterol.

You can find tofu in the produce section of the supermarket. There are a variety of styles to choose from.

* *Extra-firm tofu is perfect for slicing, dicing, and stir-frying. It holds together for broiling, baking, and boiling. This variety provides more protein than any other style of tofu.*

* *Firm tofu can also be used for slicing, dicing, and pan-frying. It is of a lighter consistency than extra-firm.*

* *Soft tofu is great to use in sauces, soups, and salads.*

* *Silken tofu is great to use in soups, desserts, and beverages. It has a smooth, delicate, and custard-like texture.*

Flavored tofu is also available, but these varieties contain a lot of sodium. Since tofu acts like a sponge, your best bet is to mix tofu with garlic, scallions, low-sodium sauces, olive oil and other flavorful ingredients that are absorbed easily. Substitute tofu for chicken or beef in traditional recipes like chili, pasta, or stir-fry. Whip up substitutes for cream cheese or cottage cheese with tofu. Blend tofu with miso in a food processor for a variety of spreads and dips!

To keep tofu fresh, store it in the refrigerator submerged in water and change the water daily. Your tofu will last 7 to 10 days after it has been opened. You can also freeze tofu. Take it out of its package and wrap it up in something air tight. Tofu that has been frozen is darker in color and has a chewy texture. You can keep it frozen up to 5 months. Spoiled tofu should be immediately thrown away! You can detect spoiled tofu by its sour smell, or by a cloudy appearance in the water. Other soybean based foods include tempeh, soy milk, miso (fermented soybean paste), and edamame (green vegetable soybeans).

Chapter 4

♦ ♦ ❖ ♦ ♦ ❖ ♦ ♦ ❖ ♦ ♦ ❖ ♦ ♦ ❖ ♦ ♦ ❖ ♦ ♦

Planning a Nutritious Day

Eating well means enjoying a variety of food—and so does eating to stay well. Variety is important because no one food has all the nutrients, and other substances that your heart, as well as the rest of your body, requires to function. It is better to eat a variety of foods than to rely on supplements for adequate nutrition. Many foods have nutrients that work with each other to enhance their utilization. An example of this is milk. It contains calcium, vitamin D, and phosphorus, all of which are absorbed together to build strong, healthy bones. A supplement may contain calcium, but it may be lacking vitamin D or phosphorus, preventing the calcium from being used to its fullest potential. Following a well-balanced eating plan is the best way to ensure that you look great on the inside as well as the out!

The nutrient list that accompanies the recipes in this collection will help you do just that. Nutrients vital for good heart health are noted at the end of each recipe. Let this list assist you in obtaining the recommended daily total intakes of these critical nutrients. The recommended daily intakes for healthy adults are discussed below. Keep in mind that your nutrient needs may differ if you are over-weight, have heart disease, high blood pressure, high cholesterol, diabetes, or a number of other health conditions. If health issues apply, check with your physician or a registered dietitian to determine what levels are optimal for you.

Daily calorie and nutrient intakes:

Calories. Consume enough to achieve and maintain a healthy weight. A calorie is a unit of energy, not a nutrient. The amount that's best for you depends largely on your height, weight, and activity level. You'll also need to consider whether or not you would like to lose weight. One pound is equivalent to 3500 calories. Slimming your calorie needs by 500 per day will result in a weight loss of one pound per week. Other factors that affect your calorie needs include how physically active you are and your age. Calories are the source of energy our bodies use to perform tasks; the more active you are, the more calories you will burn. Additionally, middle-aged and older adults tend to need fewer calories than their younger counterparts. General daily calorie and nutrient guidelines are as follows:

* *1,600 calories*   *For young children (ages 2 to 6), women, and some older adults*

* *2,200 calories*   *For older children, teenage girls, active women, and most men*

* *2,800 calories*   *For teenage boys and active men*

Nutrients. Substances necessary for growth, normal body functioning and maintaining life. Daily guidelines for those greatly impacting heart health are as follows:

* *Total fat*   *No more than 30 percent of daily calories*

* *Saturated fat*   *Less than 10 percent of daily calories*

* *Cholesterol*   *Less than 300 milligrams per day*

* *Fiber*   *25 to 30 grams per day*

* *Protein*   *10 to 35 percent of daily calories*

* *Carbohydrates*   *45 to 65 percent of daily calories*

* *Sodium*   *No more than 2,400 milligrams per day*

To calculate percent of daily calories, it's important to know that protein and carbohydrate have 4 calories per gram, while fat has 9 calories per gram. For example, if you eat 2,000 calories a day, your daily intake should be no more than 67 grams of total fat (2000 calories X 30% = 600 calories from fat, then divide the 600 calories from fat by 9 to convert it into grams of total fat) and no more than 22 grams of saturated fat. A desirable carbohydrate intake for a person consuming 2,000 calories daily is 225 to 325 grams (2000 calories X 45% to 65% = 900 to 1300 calories from carbohydrate. Divide these by 4 and you get 225 to 325 grams daily). Using the same calculating method you will find that an ideal protein intake for a 2,000 calorie diet is 50 to 175 grams daily.

Use these guidelines as just that, guidelines! Remember the goal is to build a nutritious diet from nutritious meals. Not every dish or food needs to be low in fat and/or calories. Keep your sights set on an overall healthy eating pattern.

Sample Breakfasts

(Approximately 200 to 400 calories)

Eating breakfast will energize your mind and body in the morning. Whether you choose a blender shake or an egg omelet on whole wheat toast, a hearty breakfast will prevent you from overindulging at later meals.

1 low-fat whole grain waffle   Total calories: 330
(Try Eggo™ or Go Lean Kashi™ varieties)
1 Tbsp light syrup (sugar-free)
1 small banana
½ cup calcium fortified orange juice

½ cup whole grain cereal   Total calories: 320
(Choose a cereal with > 2 grams fiber/serving)
8 oz skim milk/Skim Plus™/1% milk,
1 small banana

1 packet of instant oatmeal   Total calories: 190
1 piece of fruit

12 oz non-fat latte   Total: 400 calories
½ whole wheat bagel (scooped out)
1 tsp nut butter with sliced banana

whole wheat bagel/english muffin   Total: 260 calories
1 tsp margarine/butter
1 tsp jelly

gourmet egg substitute omelet: Total: 240 calories
½ cup egg substitute
1 cup chopped veggies (scallion, onion,
   tomatoes, peppers, mushrooms)
1 tsp canola/olive oil (to sauté the vegetables)
1 whole wheat tortilla or 1 slice whole grain toast

1 cup 1% cottage cheese   Total: 250 calories
½ cup fruit salad or small piece of fruit

1 egg/1 slice of ham or 2 strips of soy bacon   Total: 270 calories
on whole wheat English muffin

grilled cheese on pita bread   Total: 280 calories
1 mini whole wheat pita
¼ cup low-fat shredded cheese
2 Tbsp tomato sauce
tomato slices
garlic/onion powder for seasoning

Watch out for bakery bagels—the calories add up quickly. Most bagels weigh 5 oz. At 80 calories per ounce, that translates into a 400 calorie bagel without spread! Instead, choose *high-quality* carbs in sensible portions, such as whole wheat varieties, pumpernickel, or rye. Lender's bagels or Thomas English muffins count as more sensible servings.

Sample Recipes

Breakfast Quesadilla

2 tsp olive oil

1 cup chopped scallions, garlic, tomatoes, red/green/yellow peppers, mushrooms

1 16 oz package of firm tofu

1 cup of canned organic black beans

¼ cup fat-free shredded cheese

4 100% 6" whole wheat tortillas

4 Tbsp salsa

---

1. Heat olive oil in skillet over medium heat.

2. Sauté vegetables.

3. Add tofu and beans.

4. Melt cheese.

5. Spoon mixture into tortillas. Divide evenly.

6. Add salsa.

NUTRITIONAL FACTS	
CALORIES:	229.15KCALS
PROTEIN:	11.71G
CARBS:	28.91G
TOTAL FAT:	6.29G
SAT FAT:	1.27G
CHOLESTEROL:	5.00MG
SODIUM: 381.97MG	
FIBER: 13.07G	
CALCIUM: 180.52MG	
POTASSIUM: 118.90MG	
YIELD:	4 SERVINGS
SERVING SIZE: 1 TORTILLA WITH FILLING (4 OZ. TOFU, 2 TBSP CHEESE, ⅓ CUP BEANS, 1 TBSP SALSA, ¼ CUP VEGETABLES)	

Start your day with a balanced breakfast. This recipe is packed with fiber, making it a healthier alternative to a bagel with cream cheese. Tofu acts like a sponge, absorbing the natural flavor of the vegetables (the scallion is the key ingredient!) and is a good source of soy protein. Tofu is usually found in the produce section of grocery stores. Eden organic beans only contain 15 mg sodium per ½ cup serving.

Try eating every 3 to 5 hours to help rebound hunger pangs.

Mid-morning snack ideas:	
2 oz canned salmon in water wrapped in lettuce 1 Tbsp reduced fat mayo	Total: 205 calories
4 Tbsp Hummus ½ to 1 cup carrot / celery sticks	Total: 205 calories

Berry and Banana Smoothie

1 cup of calcium-fortified fat-free choco-
late-vanilla swirl frozen yogurt
(The food label should read >20% Daily
Value for calcium)
1 cup of frozen berries
1 banana sliced
¾ cup Skim Plus™/Fat-free Plus Milk™
(fat-free milk with a thick flavor)

---

1. Pour ingredients in blender.
2. Blend until smooth (approximately
1 minute).

NUTRITIONAL FACTS	
CALORIES:	385.79KCALS
PROTEIN:	10.55G
CARBS:	83.98G
TOTAL FAT:	2.59G
SAT FAT:	1.22G
CHOLESTEROL:	10.00MG
SODIUM:	209.90MG
FIBER:	4.58G
CALCIUM:	313.31MG
POTASSIUM:	957.08MG
YIELD:	4 SERVINGS
SERVING SIZE:	1 CUP

This recipe is an easy way to start your day with a power breakfast. The nutrients in frozen fruit are well preserved, enabling you to enjoy fruits when they are not in season or freshly available.

Don't Ignore Portion Size

Did you know that a cup is about the size of a tennis ball? That a heaping teaspoon is equal to a level tablespoon and that three ounces of meat is about the size of a deck of cards? If you aren't careful, it's very easy to misjudge how much food you are actually taking in.

Often items are packaged in what appears to be a single serving. Glancing at the portion size on the food label may tell you differently. For example, a vending machine bag containing eight cookies may indicate that the serving size is actually four cookies and the servings per package are two. Because all of the nutrition information noted on the label applies to the specific portion size listed, you are actually getting two times the nutrient (including calorie) amount noted if the entire package is eaten.

Huge portions served by restaurants further complicate things. As a country, we have learned to accept these portions as the norm, making it easy to pile on unwanted pounds unknowingly. The recipes in this collection are designed to teach you to eat sensibly and provide portions that will satisfy you.

A Pyramid of Healthy Foods

We've talked about heart disease risk factors and just how greatly what and how much you eat influences them. We've talked about how to read a food label and how to interpret the claims seen on them. Furthermore, you can now evaluate specific food items to determine if they are heart-healthy. But, how do you mold all of this into a well-balanced eating plan? By using the Food Guide Pyramid developed by the U.S. Department of Agriculture.

This pyramid is designed to show you groups of food that make up a nutritious diet. The base of the pyramid forms the foundation for good nutrition and depicts the foods that you should eat most often. As you go up the pyramid, the recommended number of servings from each group represented decrease. Choosing the correct amount of servings in the proper portion ensures that you will receive the nutrients that your body requires without consuming too much fat, saturated fat, cholesterol, sodium, sugar, or alcohol. This plan also controls for calories, thereby helping you take charge of your weight.

How To Use the Food Guide Pyramid: A Guide To Daily Food Choices

6 to 11 SERVINGS

Bread, Cereal Rice, and Pasta Group (especially whole grains)
   1 slice bread
   1 cup of ready-to-eat cereal
   ½ cup cooked cereal, rice, or pasta

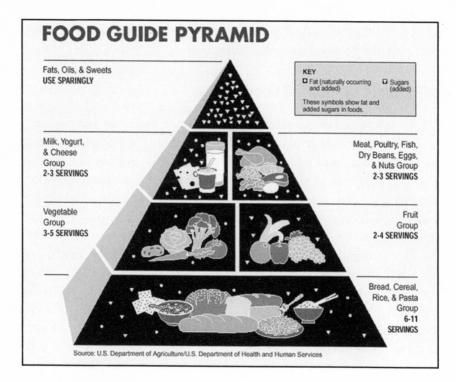

FOOD GUIDE PYRAMID

Fats, Oils, & Sweets
USE SPARINGLY

KEY
□ Fat (naturally occurring and added) □ Sugars (added)
These symbols show fat and added sugars in foods.

Milk, Yogurt, & Cheese Group
2-3 SERVINGS

Meat, Poultry, Fish, Dry Beans, Eggs, & Nuts Group
2-3 SERVINGS

Vegetable Group
3-5 SERVINGS

Fruit Group
2-4 SERVINGS

Bread, Cereal, Rice, & Pasta Group
6-11 SERVINGS

Source: U.S. Department of Agriculture/U.S. Department of Health and Human Services

2 to 4 SERVINGS

Fruit Group
1 medium apple, banana, orange, or pear
½ cup of chopped, cooked, or canned fruit
¾ cup fruit juice

2 to 3 SERVINGS

Meat, Poultry, Fish, Dry Beans, Eggs, and Nuts Group (preferably lean)
2 to 3 ounces of cooked lean meat, poultry, or fish
counts as one ounce of lean meat:
½ cup cooked dry beans, peas, and lentils
½ cup tofu
2 Tbsp peanut butter
⅓ cup of nuts
2½ oz soy burger
1 egg

3 to 5 SERVINGS

Vegetable Group
   1 cup raw leafy vegetables
   ½ cup dry beans, peas and lentils
   ½ cup other vegetables—cooked or raw
   ¾ cup vegetable juice
   (Note: dry beans, peas, and lentils can be counted as servings in either the meat and beans group or the vegetable group.)

2 to 3 SERVINGS

Milk, Yogurt, and Cheese Group (preferably fat-free or low-fat)
   1 cup milk or yogurt
   1½ oz natural cheese (such as Cheddar)
   2 oz processed cheese (such as American)

USE SPARINGLY

Fats, Oils, and Sweets
   ⅛ avocado
   1 Tbsp salad dressing
   1 Tbsp cream cheese
   1 tsp butter, oil, margarine, or mayonnaise
   10 peanuts
   ½ cup ice cream
   1 small cupcake or muffin
   2 small cookies

This group sits at the top of the pyramid, indicating that your needs are very little from this category. Fat is required by your body for some things like the absorption of Vitamins A, D, E, and K. Too much fat, as you know, can be harmful to your body. Sweets can give you quick energy because they are carbohydrates but often provide little in the way of nutrients and are frequently high in calories. Use the following table to get a better idea of the correct number of servings you should consume according to your calorie intake.

HOW TO USE THE FOOD GUIDE PYRAMID

What counts as a serving?	1600 calories*	2200 calories*	2800 calories*
Bread, Cereal, Rice and Pasta group	6	9	11
• 1 slice of bread			
• About 1 cup of ready-to-eat cereal			
• 1/2 cup cooked cereal, rice, or pasta			
Vegetable Group	3	4	5
• 1 cup raw leafy vegetables			
• 1/2 cup other vegetables—cooked or raw			
• 3/4 cup vegetable juice			
Fruit Group	2	3	4
• 1 medium apple, banana, orange, pear			
• 1/2 cup chopped, cooked, or canned fruit			
• 3/4 cup fruit juice			
Milk, Yogurt, and Cheese Group	2 or 3**	2 or 3**	2 or 3**
(preferably fat-free or low-fat)			
• 1 cup of milk••• or yogurt			
• 1 1/2 oz natural cheese (such as Cheddar)			
• 2 oz processed cheese (such as American)			
Meat, Poultry, Fish, Dry Beans, Eggs, and	2 (5 oz total)	2 (6 oz total)	3 (7 oz total)
Nuts Group (preferably lean or low-fat)			
• 2 to 3 oz cooked lean meat, poultry, or fish			

These count as 1 oz of meat:
• 1/2 cup cooked dry beans or tofu
• 2 1/2 oz soyburger
• 1 egg
• 2 Tbsp peanut butter
• 1/3 cup of nuts

*Recommended number of servings depends on your calorie needs:
• 1600 calories is about right for children ages 2 to 6 years.
• 2200 calories is about right for children over 6, teen girl s, active women, and many sedentary men.
• 2800 calories is about right for teen boys and active men.

**Children and teens ages 9 to 18 years and adults over age 50 need 3 servings daily; others need 2 servings daily.

***This includes lactose-free and lactose-reduced milk products. Soy-based beverages with added calcium are an option for those who prefer a non-dairy source of calcium.

Note: Many of the serving sizes given above are smaller than those on the Nutrition Facts Label. For example, 1 serving of cooked cereal, rice, or pasta is 1 cup for the label, but only 1/2 cup for the Pyramid.

Keeping the "Heart" in Old Family Favorites

Some of the most memorable dining experiences have involved recipes passed on from generation to generation. Unfortunately, these recipes are often laden with fat and salt. However, there is no need to give up those too rich favorite family recipes. With a few minor substitutions, you can retain the "heart and soul" of the dish without sacrificing flavor or health.

General Substitutions

Milk/Cream/Sour Cream

* Cook with low-fat (1 percent fat) or fat-free milk, instead of whole milk or cream. You may also use nonfat dry or nonfat evaporated milk.
* Instead of sour cream, use plain fat-free (or low-fat) yogurt or sour cream. You can also blend 1 cup of low-fat, unsalted cottage cheese with 1 Tbsp of fat-free milk and 2 tsp of lemon juice.

Spices/Flavorings

* Use a variety of herbs and spices in place of salt. See the upcoming section titled "making mealtimes spicy" for specific ideas.
* Use sodium-free salt substitute. (Do not use light salt, it contains sodium and studies have shown that people just sprinkle on more in order to get the same taste and thus the same amount of sodium as regular salt.)
* Use low-sodium bouillon and broths, in lieu of the regular varieties.
* Use a small amount of skinless smoked turkey breast, instead of fatback—fat from the back of a pig, often used in Southern cooking, to lower the fat content but retain taste.
* Use skinless chicken thighs, instead of neck bones, to season.

Oils/Butter/Lard

* Use nonstick cooking oil spray for stir-frying or sautéing to lower the fat content and calories.
* Use a small amount of vegetable oil, instead of lard, butter, or other fats that are hard at room temperature.
* In general, diet margarines are not well suited for baking. Instead, use spreads containing heart-healthy plant sterols and plant stanols to cut saturated fat. You can also use regular soft margarine made with vegetable oil.
* Choose margarines that list liquid vegetable oil as their first ingredient on the food label.

Eggs

* In baking use ¼ cup of egg substitute, instead of 1 whole egg.
* You may also use 3 egg whites and 1 egg yolk, instead of 2 whole eggs.

For Meats and Poultry

* Choose a lean cut of meat and remove any visible fat.
* Remove the skin from chicken and other poultry before cooking.
* Purchase extra lean ground beef such as ground round or use ground turkey or chicken breast.
* Use turkey sausage or vegetarian sausage instead of Chorizo sausage.

For Sandwiches and Salads

* In salads and sandwiches, use fat-free or low-fat dressing, yogurt, or mayonnaise, instead of regular versions.
* To make a salad dressing, use equal parts water and vinegar, and half as much oil.
* Garnish salads with fruits and vegetables.

For Soups and Stews

* Prepare broths, soups, and stews in advance and chill them. Before reheating, lift off the hardened fat that has formed at the surface. By doing this, you will remove much of the fat. If you're short on time, you may also float several ice cubes on the surface of the warm liquid to harden the fat instead of refrigeration.
* Use cooking spray, water, or stock to sauté onion for flavoring stews, soups, and sauces.
* Instead of Ramen noodles use whole-grain pasta, rice, or barley.

For Breads

* To make muffins, quick breads, or biscuits, use no more than 1 to 2 Tbsp of fat (lard, butter, margarine, or oil) for each cup of flour.
* When preparing muffins or quick breads, use three ripe, very well mashed bananas instead of ½ cup of butter or oil. You can also substitute a cup of applesauce for a cup of butter, margarine, oil, or shortening. This reduces both saturated fat and calories.

For Desserts

* To make a pie crust, use only ½ cup margarine for every 2 cups flour.
* For chocolate desserts, use 3 Tbsp of cocoa, instead of 1 oz of baking chocolate. If fat is needed to replace what was in the chocolate, add 1 Tbsp or less of vegetable oil.
* To make cakes and soft-drop cookies, use no more than 2 Tbsp of fat for each cup of flour.

Making Mealtime Spicy

Less fat? Less salt? How do you preserve the taste? It's easy if you flavor with spices and herbs. Although these terms are used interchangeably, spices are ground seeds, flowers, or bark, while herbs are leaves. If you are unsure whether a particular herb or spice will enhance a food, first smell and taste the herb that you are considering. Then determine if the herb or spice complements the aroma of what's on the stove. Fresh herbs last about a week in the refrigerator if you wrap the stems in a moist paper towel and then put them in a zip lock bag. When using fresh herbs, use ⅔ more than you would if the herb was dried.

Use the following table to assist you in enhancing the flavor of a specific food:

Meat, Poultry, and Fish

Beef.	Basil, bay leaf, cayenne pepper, cloves, dill, ginger, garlic powder, ground mustard, marjoram, nutmeg, onion powder, oregano, paprika, parsley, pepper, rosemary, sage, tarragon, thyme
Lamb.	Cinnamon, cloves, cumin, curry powder, garlic, mint, oregano, rosemary, and sage
Pork.	Cloves, cumin, garlic, nutmeg, onion powder, oregano, pepper, sage
Veal.	Bay leaf, curry powder, ginger, marjoram, oregano
Poultry.	Basil, cayenne pepper, cinnamon, dill, garlic powder, ginger, ground mustard, marjoram, nutmeg, onion powder, oregano, paprika, parsley, rosemary, sage, tarragon, thyme
Fish.	Bay leaf, cayenne pepper, curry powder, dill, ginger, ground mustard, lemon juice, marjoram, onion powder, oregano, paprika, parsley, pepper, rosemary, tarragon, thyme

Vegetables

Carrots.	Cinnamon, cloves, marjoram, nutmeg, rosemary, sage
Corn.	Cumin, curry powder, onion powder, paprika, parsley
Green beans.	Dill, curry powder, lemon juice, marjoram, oregano, tarragon, thyme
Greens.	Onion powder, ground mustard. pepper
Peas.	Ginger, marjoram, onion powder, parsley, sage
Potatoes.	Dill, garlic, onion powder, paprika, parsley, sage
Summer squash.	Cloves, curry powder, marjoram, nutmeg, rosemary, sage
Winter squash.	Cinnamon, ginger, nutmeg, onion powder
Tomatoes.	Basil, bay leaf, dill, marjoram, onion powder, oregano, parsley, pepper

Chapter 5

♦ ♦ ❖ ♦ ♦ ❖ ♦ ♦ ❖ ♦ ♦ ❖ ♦ ♦ ❖ ♦ ♦ ❖ ♦ ♦

Fiber, Salt, and Vitamins

Fast Facts on Fiber, Fat, and Salt

We've been promoting whole grains. We've told you to cut down on fat and salt. You've heard that there are different kinds of fiber and you've heard that there are good and bad fats. So... what are the differences and what are the benefits? Read on!

Fiber—Why Does It Matter, and What Is It Anyway?

Why the strong emphasis on fiber? Because it's vital for good health! A wealth of research suggests that fiber helps to reduce LDL (bad) cholesterol levels, thereby lowering your risk of heart disease. It also seems to relieve constipation and decrease the symptoms of both diverticulosis and irritable bowel syndrome. Dietary fiber provides bulk without calories causing you to feel full on fewer calories. This is a real bonus if weight loss is one of your goals! Additionally, it has been linked to cancer prevention, particularly colon and breast cancer. High fiber diets even seem to help control blood sugar. This is especially important if you have diabetes or are at risk of developing the disease.

So what is this stuff? Fiber is a component in plants that your body is unable to digest or absorb. Because fiber never enters your bloodstream, it is not considered a nutrient. There are two main types of fiber—soluble (also called "viscous") and insoluble. While both have health benefits, only soluble fiber reduces the risk of heart disease.

The key ingredient needed by your body to make cholesterol is fat. In the digestive tract, soluble fiber mixes with liquid and binds to fatty substances. They are then removed from the body. If fat has been removed from the body, then less fat is available to make cholesterol with. Soluble fiber also prolongs the time it takes for the stomach to empty. As a result, sugar is released and absorbed more slowly. This helps to control blood sugar levels. Insoluble fiber (often called "roughage") passes through the digestive tract largely intact. This fiber helps the colon function properly promoting regular bowel movements and preventing constipation. It also moves toxic waste through the colon rapidly and helps to keep colon acidity at the level it should be, reducing cancer risk.

Ideally, total fiber intake should be about 25 to 30 grams daily with a minimum of 5 to 10 grams coming from soluble fiber. Many foods contain both soluble and insoluble fiber. Generally, fruits have more soluble fiber and vegetables are richer in insoluble fiber. The table below outlines the best food sources for each of these types of fiber.

Good Food Sources of Soluble Fiber

Whole grain cereals and seeds. Barley; oatmeal; oat bran; whole-wheat products such as psyllium seeds (ground) wheat oat, corn bran, flax seed

Fruits. Apples (with the skin); bananas; pears; blackberries; oranges; grapefruits; nectarines; peaches; pears; plums; prunes

Legumes. Black, kidney, lima, navy, northern, yellow, green, and pinto beans; yellow, green, and orange lentils and orange lentils; chickpeas and black-eyed peas

Vegetables. Broccoli; brussel sprouts; carrots; green beans; cauliflower; potatoes (with their skin)

10 Tip Plan to Boost Your Fiber Intake

1. Plan vegetable based meals. Add vegetables to sandwiches, pizza, and pasta. Tip: use the plate method to portion your food. ¼ portion starch (includes starchy vegetables such as corn, peas, squash, potatoes with skin), ¼ portion lean protein, and ½ should be non-starchy vegetables. If you are eating a low-fat frozen dinner and still feel hungry, prepare vegetables as a side dish.

2. Switch from white flour products to wheat flour products. Make sure the first ingredient on the food label is 100% whole wheat flour, not enriched wheat flour. You can also find whole grain breads and crackers made from rye and oats. Thomas's English muffins or Lenders bagels come in whole-wheat varieties and are sensibly sized compared to a jumbo bakery bagel! Eating out? Order brown rice instead of white rice at Chinese restaurants. You can also request brown-rice sushi at some Japanese restaurants.

3. Choose fruit over fruit juice. Eat fruit with edible seeds such as kiwi, blueberries, raspberries, and figs.

4. Boost your bean intake! Eat bean-based soups. Add black beans, kidney beans, peas, and lentils to salads, chile, and burritos Tip: eat fresh or frozen beans. If you select a canned variety, go with a "No salt added" product such as Eden Organic beans.

5. Movie watching snacks: baby carrots, celery, and sliced cucumbers dipped in hummus (the fiber in hummus comes from ground chickpeas), or dried fruit, mixed with unsalted fat-free popcorn and almonds, soy nuts, and sunflower seeds.

6. Eat whole-wheat pasta dishes. The fiber content will add bulk to your diet, leaving you less likely to consume large quantities.

7. Make a "very veggie" lasagna using thick strips of squash and zucchini as a substitute for noodles. Layer additional vegetables (spinach, tomatoes, carrots, pepper, onions, or broccoli) with low-sodium tomato sauce in between zucchini and squash strips.

8. Microwave frozen edamame (soy beans that resemble pea pods) for a quick snack. This is a great finger food!

9. Include the skins in mashed potatoes.

10. Top a whole grain cereal with fresh fruit slices (a natural sweetener packed with nutrients). Select an unsweetened cereal to eliminate added sugar and calories from your diet.

If you are trying to lose weight, remember to use the exchange lists or the Food Guide Pyramid as guidelines for portion control.

Sample Recipe:

Nature's Harvest Sandwich

1 whole wheat English muffin or 2 slices
   of 100% whole wheat bread
1 Tbsp Dijon mustard
1 cup of raw vegetables (alfalfa sprouts,
   tomatoes, shredded carrots, cucumbers,
   spinach leaves)
¼ cup avocado slices
1 boiled egg, yolk removed

---

1. Spread mustard on each English muffin
   half.
2. Layer with vegetables and avocado.
3. Top with egg whites.

NUTRITIONAL FACTS	
CALORIES:	228.44KCALS
PROTEIN:	11.14G
CARBS:	32.44G
TOTAL FAT:	6.84G
SAT FAT:	1.08G
CHOLESTEROL:	0.00MG
SODIUM:	299.33MG
FIBER:	6.47G
CALCIUM:	126.49MG
POTASSIUM:	377.43MG
YIELD:	1 SERVING
SERVING SIZE:	1 SANDWICH

Did you know the top 4 vegetables consumed by Americans are tomatoes in the form of ketchup, potatoes in the form of French fries, iceberg lettuce, and onions? This recipe is a healthy way to increase fiber in a sandwich. The avocado is a good source of monounsaturated fat. The egg whites add some protein to the meal.

Salt—How Can I Reduce the Amount of Salt I Eat?

You are aware that reducing salt in the diet can prevent high blood pressure in people at risk for the disease. People most likely to be sensitive to salt (sodium chloride) include: those of African descent, people with kidney disease, people with a family history of high blood pressure, and those over age 50. Most Americans eat too much salt, exceeding the American Heart Association's recommendations of a maximum of 2400 mg of sodium daily. Although getting rid of the salt shaker will help, only about 15 percent of sodium is consumed via table salt. Nearly 75 percent of the salt in our diet comes from processed foods. The remaining 10 percent is naturally present in the foods that we eat.

If you're trying to reduce your intake of salt and sodium, try choosing low-sodium, or reduced sodium, or no salt added versions of foods and condiments whenever available. You should use fresh, frozen, or canned "with no salt added" vegetables, as well as fresh poultry, fish, and lean meat. Stay away from salty or smoked meats such as hot dogs, lunch meats, ham, sausage, bacon, smoked salmon, and canned tuna.

Foods packed in brine such as pickles, pickled vegetables, olives, and sauerkraut should be eaten rarely, and sauce mixes, canned, and instant soups should be used sparingly. Limit high sodium condiments including horseradish, catsup, and barbeque sauce. Even the lower sodium versions of soy sauce and teriyaki sauce contain a tremendous amount of sodium.

Salt itself is a large source of sodium. Try cooking rice, pasta, and hot cereals without salt. Instant or flavored rice, pasta, and cereal mixes typically have added salt, so use them rarely. Be sure to choose breakfast cereals that contain less than 20 percent of your daily value for sodium. Also avoid the hidden sodium on ingredient labels. It is listed as monosodium glutamate (MSG) and disodium phosphate.

Make sure your "convenience" foods are as low in sodium as possible. Frozen dinners should contain less than 800 mg of sodium. Cut back on mixed dishes such as pizza, packaged mixes, and salad dressings. If you use canned foods, such as tuna, rinse them to remove some of the sodium.

When you cook and at the table, flavor your food with herbs, spices, lemon, lime, vinegar, or salt-free seasoning blends. Try one new herb or spice in a recipe each week. Be careful, however, some seasoning blends, such as lemon pepper, contain a significant amount of sodium. Be sure to check the ingredient list on all seasoning blends. Also, try using half as much salt in a recipe than it suggests. (The recipes in this book have already been adjusted.)

Be Good to Your Body with "B" vitamins

Why are B vitamins important for heart health?

Take a moment to think about a typical morning. It requires energy to shower, get dressed, prepare breakfast, read the newspaper, and

Sample Recipe:

Sloppy Joe

1   16 oz package of 100% whole wheat
     penne pasta
1   Tbsp olive oil
2   garlic cloves, minced
1   lb extra lean ground turkey
     pepper to taste
1   cup Healthy Choice™ tomato sauce
8   Tbsp parmesan cheese

NUTRITIONAL FACTS	
CALORIES:	577.82KCALS
PROTEIN:	47.26G
CARBS:	69.72G
TOTAL FAT:	10.57G
SAT FAT:	3.32G
CHOLESTEROL:	58.38MG
SODIUM:	326.39MG
FIBER:	12.25G
CALCIUM:	212.00MG
POTASSIUM:	13.38MG
YIELD:	4 SERVINGS
SERVING SIZE:	1 CUP PASTA, 4 OUNCES TURKEY, ¼ CUP SAUCE, 2 TBSP PARMESAN CHEESE

1. Prepare pasta according to package directions.
2. Heat olive oil in skillet over medium-high heat. Sauté garlic.
3. Season the turkey with pepper. Add to skillet and cook through until meat is browned.
4. Add sauce on turkey. Serve over pasta. Sprinkle with parmesan cheese.

The whole wheat pasta adds bulk to this entree and is a simple way to sneak in dietary fiber. The extra lean turkey is an excellent source of protein with very little saturated fat. Healthy Choice sauce is preferable because it is lower in sodium than a regular Sloppy Joe sauce.

---

plan activities for the day. In order to achieve these tasks, your body needs an ongoing source of fuel. All vitamins play an important role in keeping our bodies running smoothly, especially the B-complex vitamins. These eight vitamins help break down the carbohydrates, proteins, and fats from your diet into energy.

Three B's worth knowing for their heart-healthy role include vitamin B-9 (folic acid), vitamin B6, and vitamin B12. If you get too little folic acid, an amino acid called homocysteine can accumulate in your blood. Homocysteine can potentially harm cells that line the heart and blood vessels. Men have higher homocyteine levels than women. Aging can cause homocysteine to rise. High levels of homocysteine may also be due to homocytinuria, a rare genetic disorder that occurs when the liver is unable to clear homocysteine from the body. Folic acid works with B6 and B12 to metabolize homocysteine and bring blood levels down to a safe range. If these vitamins are in short supply, homocysteine levels can build up (high is considered above 10 to 12 micromoles per liter), causing plaque formation around the arteries that can eventually lead to a heart attack.

B vitamins are water soluble, which means they are easily broken down and absorbed by the body. It also means that you need an ongoing supply, because the kidneys excrete most of what your body doesn't immediately use.

Recipe and Snack Ideas to Boost Your Intake of B Vitamins

Strawberries on a Cloud

2 cantaloupes, divided

8 Tbsp fat-free cool whip or plain fat-free yogurt

2 cups of sliced strawberries

1. Scoop out cantaloupe seeds.
2. Spoon 2 Tbsp of cool whip onto each cantaloupe half
3. Top with strawberries. Enjoy!

The cantaloupe bowl topped with strawberries on a cloud of cool whip makes this recipe simple, delicious, and a sweet way to get folic acid.

NUTRITIONAL FACTS	
CALORIES:	110.43KCALS
PROTEIN:	2.96G
CARBS:	24.60G
TOTAL FAT:	1.40G
SAT FAT:	0.48G
CHOLESTEROL:	2.19MG
SODIUM:	29.93MG
FIBER:	3.51G
CALCIUM:	53.59MG
POTASSIUM:	834.71MG
YIELD:	4 SERVINGS
SERVING SIZE: 1 CANTALOUPE HALF, 2 TBSP COOL WHIP, ½ CUP STRAWBERRIES	

Trail Mix Ideas

Note: use a maximum of one ounce of nuts per serving of trail mix. The following equal one ounce: 24 almonds, 18 medium cashews,

How to get your daily dose of B vitamins through diet:

Vitamin B-9/ Folic acid (synthetic form) / **Folate** (natural form in foods)
Role: Folate is important in red blood cell formation, protein metabolism, growth and cell division. It's also important during pregnancy for the developing fetus.
Recommended Dietary Allowance for Adults: 400 mcg/day to help protect arteries
Maximum daily intake: 1,000 mcg/day

Heart-healthy food sources include citrus fruits, dark leafy green, nuts, beans, and fortified grain products. Eight medium strawberries (provide 20% of your Daily Value) or five stalks of asparagus (provides 30% of your Daily Value) are excellent sources of folic acid. Other good sources include cantaloupe, raspberries, oranges, spinach, broccoli, and leaf lettuce. A sure way to get your daily needs of folic acid is to take a multivitamin, but foods offer the benefit of delicious flavor and supply a variety of nutrients.

In 1998, the FDA required that folic acid be added to enriched grained-foods such as bread, pasta, and rice. In addition, the FDA authorized ready-to-eat cereals to be fully fortified up to 100% of the Daily Value of folic acid. By eating a highly fortified cereal with low-fat milk and berries for breakfast, you can easily get a healthy dose of folic acid.

Vitamin B-6:
Role: Vitamin B-6 is essential for protein metabolism, energy production, and brain function. It aids in the formation of several hormones, such as serotonin which regulates sleep and mood.
Recommended Dietary Allowance for Adults: 1.3 mg/dy
Ages 51 or older- Men:1.7 mg/day; Women: 1.5 mg/day
Maximum daily intake: 100 mg/day

Heart-healthy food sources include skinless chicken, salmon, swordfish, pork loin, soybeans, oats, whole grain products, nuts, seeds, bananas, egg substitutes, and avocados.

Vitamin B12
Role: Vitamin B-12 plays an essential role in red blood cell formation, cell metabolism, and nerve function. An adequate supply is

needed to support proper digestion and produce energy from fat and sugar.

Recommended Dietary Allowance for Adults: 2.4 mcg/day
Maximum daily intake: unknown

Heart-healthy food sources include 3 oz of lean sirloin, fish, shellfish, poultry, eggs/egg substitutes, and low-fat dairy products. Fortified breakfast cereals may also contain B-12. Note: Vegetarians who eliminate all animal foods from their diet may benefit from a vitamin B-12 supplement. If you're over age 50, your body is less able to absorb vitamin B-12 from animal foods, and you may benefit from fortified foods or supplements.

There is still not enough evidence to confirm a true cause-and-effect relationship between homocysteine and heart disease. Homocyteine may just be a traveler of vascular disease rather than a cause of it. Further scientific research is needed to determine if treating high homocysteine levels can effectively reduce the risk of cardiac disease. Fortunately, eating a heart-healthy diet that includes good sources of B vitamins is a harmless recommendation.

12 hazelnuts, 8 medium Brazil nuts, 35 unsalted peanuts, 15 pecan halves, and 14 English walnut halves. (1 oz of nuts = 160–200 calories.)

Small snack: ½ cup serving

Cereal combo: Mix Cheerios™ and Whole-Grain Chex™ with dried fruit, dried cranberries, dry roasted soy nuts, and fat-free granola.

Rain forest munch: Mix the fruits of the rain forest in a snack sized baggie: Dried pineapple and papaya pieces, cashews, and chocolate soy nuts.

Bird seed: Mix sunflower seeds, pumpkin seeds, raisins, peanuts, unsalted whole wheat pretzels, and dried dates.

Omega mix: Uncle Sam's Flax cereal, soy crisps, and honey roasted almond slivers.

Sweet treat: raisins, dried apricots, dried apple pieces, bran flakes, and Kashi™ Heart to Heart cereal.

Note: If you wish to try a different cereal, remember that any cereal with at least 3 grams of fiber per serving, and less than 8 grams of sugar per serving is a healthy choice. Fortified cereals and nuts are a great way to get B vitamins!

Chapter 6

◆ ◆ ❖ ◆ ◆ ❖ ◆ ◆ ❖ ◆ ◆ ❖ ◆ ◆ ❖ ◆ ◆ ❖ ◆ ◆

Fats

Fat—Isn't It Always Bad for You?

No! Fat benefits our bodies in various ways. It is an energy source for our body. Also, without fat, certain vitamins including A, D, E, and K cannot be absorbed. When the fat that you eat is converted into fatty tissue it acts as an insulator, keeping our bodies warm. Fatty tissue also serves as a cushion, protecting our vital organs from injury. There are several different types of fat. Knowing which ones raise LDL (bad) blood cholesterol is the first step in lowering your risk of heart disease. Dietary cholesterol, saturated fat, and trans-fats all raise bad blood cholesterol levels. Polyunsaturated and monounsaturated fats do not. Furthermore, some studies indicate that they might even lower LDL levels when the total diet is low in saturated fat. To gain a better understanding of these fats, read on.

Cholesterol is only found in foods of animal origin. The food sources with the greatest amount of cholesterol are egg yolks and organ meats. The cholesterol that you eat raises LDL cholesterol but there is a much stronger connection between LDL and the amount of saturated fat that you consume.

Saturated fat is the main dietary source of high cholesterol. This fat is usually solid at room and refrigerator temperatures.

It is found in greatest amounts in foods from animals, such as fatty cuts of meat, poultry with the skin, whole-milk dairy products, and lard. Some vegetable oils, including coconut and palm oils, also contain saturated fat.

Trans fatty acids are formed by manipulating the fat molecule during food processing. Foods high in trans-fatty acids raise blood cholesterol. Items containing large amounts of partially hydrogenated vegetable oils, including many hard margarines, shortenings, commercially fried foods, and bakery goods, all fall into this category.

Polyunsaturated fat is usually in liquid form at room and refrigerator temperatures. This fat does not increase bad blood cholesterol and may even help to lower it. Polyunsaturated fat is most prevalent in plant-based foods, including safflower, sunflower, corn, soybean, and cottonseed oils, as well as many kinds of nuts. A type of polyunsaturated fat, called an omega-3 fatty acid, is currently being studied to see if it helps guard against heart disease. Certain fish, such as salmon, tuna, and mackerel are good sources of omega-3 fatty acids.

Monounsaturated fat also may help lower blood cholesterol. Foods from plants, including olive, canola, sunflower, and peanut oils contain significant amounts of this type of fat.

Although both polyunsaturated fats and monounsaturated fats are heart-healthy, try not to overeat them or weight gain will result.

Omega-3 Fatty Acids

Omega-3 fatty acids have been promoted for their amazing health properties. Omega-3 oils alter the production of a group of biological compounds called eicosanoids, which may decrease your risk of heart disease, inflammatory processes, and certain cancers. They have been shown to exert cardio-protective effects by decreasing blood lipids (LDL cholesterol and triglycerides), decreasing blood clotting factors in the vascular system, increasing relaxation in larger arteries and blood vessels, and decreasing inflammatory processes in blood vessels. Omega-3's are polyunsaturated fats found in many oily fish. The highest ranked species of fish are Pacific herring, Atlantic herring, Pacific mackerel, Atlantic salmon, and sablefish (contain 2 or more grams of omega-3 fats for a 4 ounce serving, cooked). Other good sources of omega-3's include canned pink salmon, trout, oysters, whitefish, and sardines. Fish is also an excellent source of lean, high quality protein, assuming you do not fry it in saturated fats such as butter. Grilling, baking, poaching, or lightly sautéing in olive oil are heart-healthy ways to prepare fish. In addition, eating fat with your meals promotes satiety, making you less likely to overeat. If you don't like fish, ground flaxseed is a powerful plant source of protein and omega-3's. Flaxseed and flaxseed oil are available at health food stores and supermarkets. Flax also contains dietary fiber and lignans. Fiber adds bulk to your diet, maintains bowel regularity, and may help lower your blood cholesterol. Lignans are plant compounds that can have favorable hormone-like effects in the body. Flax has a light nutty flavor, making it a tasty addition to cereals, salads, casseroles, soups, smoothies, pasta, and baked goods.

On September 8, 2004, the Food and Drug Administration (FDA) announced that food companies could make qualified health claims on food labels concerning the heart-healthy benefits of omega-3 fatty acids. Qualified health claims are intended to keep consumers well informed of the health benefits of certain nutrients in foods. It is important to note, however, that such statements are based on limited scientific research.

The FDA limited the claims to two omega-3 acids known as eicosapentaenoic acid (EPA) and docosahexaenoic acid (DHA), which may help reduce blood triglycerides, increase HDL cholesterol, and reduce blood pressure—all actions that help lower coronary heart disease risk. Manufacturers are required to list the content of EPA and DHA in a food. Foods that exceed 13 grams of total fat or 60 mg of cholesterol per serving cannot carry the claim.

The American Heart Association recommends those with heart disease to consume 1 gram of omega-3 fatty acids per day. It is also advised to consume at least two servings of fatty fish per week, which contain both EPA and DHA. In light of warnings concerning mercury and other chemicals found in fish, the FDA announced that eating up to 12 oz of fish is safe for everyone. Since a serving size of fish is 3 to 4 oz, eating two servings per week is well below the FDA's safe limit. While flaxseed, flax oil, and flax-based omega-

---

Omega-3 fats content of foods

ALA sources:

1 Tbsp of ground flax = 1.8 grams omega-3 fats

* Ground flax is recommended over eating whole seeds because it is easier to digest.

1 Tbsp of flax oil = 8 grams of omega-3 fats

* 1 teaspoon of flax oil will meet you daily needs.

EPA and DHA sources:

1.5 ounces of fatty fish= approximately 1.5 grams of omega-3 fat (salmon, tuna, mackerel)

3-enriched eggs contain no EPA and DHA, it's a rich source of another omega-3 known as alpha-linolenic acid (ALA). ALA is an "essential" omega-3 fat, which means that it has to be obtained through your diet. However, the body can use ALA to manufacture EPA and DHA. As long as you maintain a weekly intake of 6 to 8 grams of omega-3's, your body will reap the protective benefits of these oils against coronary heart disease.

Whereas traditional health claims for food (such as the role of whole grains in reducing blood cholesterol) required years of scientific research and regulatory approval, qualified health claims were designed as a way to shorten the process. Olive oil and walnuts have also been approved for qualified health claims. For more information, visit the FDA web site at www.fda.gov.

All fats are not created equal. Trans-fatty acids have been identified as a new villain in heart disease, specifically for its artery-clogging properties. Trans-fat refers to a fatty acid that has been chemically altered by the manufacturer. These fats are often used to maintain the stability of food products, thus prolonging their shelf life. Trans-fats are primarily found in processed foods under the code ingredient "partially hydrogenated" and are frequently used in low-fat items such as cookies, crackers, granola bars, popcorn, and peanut butter to enhance flavor. They are also found in a variety of baked and fried goods along with some margarines. In fast foods, these artificial fats occur in salad dressings, buns, chicken items (chicken breasts, patties, nuggets, or tenders), french fries, milk shakes, seasonings, and croutons. In response to unfavorable health concerns related to consuming trans-fats, brand-name products have already produced a new line of trans-fat-free foods. Still, you are probably better off consuming more unsaturated fats such as olive, canola oil, and omega-3 fats.

By January 2006, the FDA requires all manufacturers to list the trans-fat content on the food label. The new label lingo allows a product to be called "trans-fat-free" if it contains less than 0.5 grams trans-fat per serving. For this reason, it is still wise to read the ingredients on the food label and trace for key words such as "hydrogenated vegetable shortening" or "partially hydrogenated oil." The easiest way to avoid excessive intake of foods containing trans-fats is by choosing whole foods over processed foods. You are better off eating the apple over the apple pie. Choose to snack on a handful of nuts and dried fruit rather than reduced fat peanut butter on low-fat crackers. In conclusion, dietary sources of saturated fat and trans-fat should be minimized.

Overview of Fats

The Facts

* *Fat is a macronutrient that supplies energy to the body—9 calories per gram*
* *Fat is needed to keep cells healthy (skin, hair, nails), regulate metabolic processes, and transport certain vitamins and minerals throughout the body.*

The fatty acids that make up the fat in food can be classified as saturated, monounsaturated, or polyunsaturated.

Figuring Your Fat

The American Heart Association recommends that no more than 300 mg of dietary cholesterol be consumed daily and keeping your

Sample recipes to boost your intake of Omega-3 fats

(1) Salmon and lettuce wraps

1 6-oz can of salmon in water
   romaine lettuce (washed and sliced into
   vertical pieces)
1 Tbsp of light mayonnaise
   diced onions (optional)

---

1. Drain salmon.
2. Mix in mayonnaise with onions.
3. Spoon mixture onto lettuce leaves. Roll
   into a wrap.

This recipe offers the nutritional bonus of
omega-3 fats. Romaine lettuce adds a nice
crunch and is a good source of vitamin C
and folate.

NUTRITIONAL FACTS

CALORIES:	99.07KCALS
PROTEIN:	12.31G
CARBS:	0.83G
TOTAL FAT:	4.78G
SAT FAT:	1.01G
CHOLESTEROL:	22.10MG
SODIUM:	74.17MG
FIBER:	0.17G
CALCIUM:	147.77MG
POTASSIUM:	170.00MG

YIELD:	3 SERVINGS

SERVING SIZE: ¼ CUP (2 OZ.)
SALMON MIXTURE WRAPPED IN
1 LETTUCE LEAF

FATTY ACID	PRIMARY FOOD SOURCES	HEALTH IMPLICATION
Saturated Fat *(generally solid at room temperature)*	Found mostly in foods from animals such as meat, poultry, and whole milk dairy products (butter, cream, milk, ice cream), vegetable oils such as coconut, palm kernel, and palm oils	* Raises blood cholesterol * When excess amounts are consumed in the diet, saturated fat is converted into body fat
Monounsaturated Fat *(usually liquid at room temperature)*	Found mostly in foods from plant origin. Olive oil, canola (rapeseed oil), peanut oil, and most nuts	* Helps reduce blood cholesterol without lowering HDL levels
Polyunsaturated Fat	*Two types include:* * Omega-6 Fatty Acid is found in plant oils such as corn, cottonseed, safflower, and sunflower oils * Omega-3 Fatty Acid is found mostly in fatty fish (salmon, tuna, mackerel, bluefish), soybeans, and flaxseed/flax oil	* Helps reduce blood cholesterol * Omega-3 Fatty Acids have been found to lower blood triglycerides and reduce blood clotting

(2) Flax French Toast

4 slices 100% whole wheat bread

1 cup egg beaters
Pam spray

8 tsp ground flaxmeal (can be purchased
at health food stores)

4 tsp sugar-free syrup
cinnamon (optional)

2 cups of fresh
strawberries/blueberries/raspberries

NUTRITIONAL FACTS	
CALORIES:	177.23KCALS
PROTEIN:	9.74G
CARBS:	26.17G
TOTAL FAT:	4.42G
SAT FAT:	0.46G
CHOLESTEROL:	0.00MG
SODIUM:	244.49MG
FIBER:	6.73G
CALCIUM:	53.01MG
POTASSIUM:	114.54MG

SERVING SIZE: 1 SLICE OF BREAD
WITH 2TSP FLAX, ½ CUP
BERRIES, 1 TSP SYRUP

---

1. Dip bread in egg beaters.
2. Heat skillet over medium heat. Lightly coat bottom of skillet with Pam spray.
3. Add bread slices. Brown each side to a light golden color.
4. Sprinkle 2 teaspoons of flax on each slice.
5. Remove from heat. Add syrup, cinnamon, and berries.

Flaxseed gives any dish a light nutty flavor. You can add it to oatmeal, smoothies, casseroles, or salads for a healthy dose of omega-3 fats. The fruit is a natural sweetener and adds an extra dose of fiber to the meal. Make sure the bread you use contains at least 3 grams of fiber per slice.

---

intake under 200 mg if you already have high cholesterol or heart disease. It also advises that no more than 30 percent of our total daily calorie intake come from fat and less than 10 percent should consist of saturated fat. These guidelines are for healthy adults. If your LDL cholesterol is over 100 mg/dl, then your total fat intake should be closer to 25 percent and your saturated fat less than seven percent of the total number of calories you consume in a day. Use the table below to translate your ideal intake into grams.

If your LDL is below 100:

1,200 calories	13 grams saturated fat	40 grams total fat
1,600 calories	18 grams saturated fat	53 grams total fat
2,000 calories	22 grams saturated fat	67 grams total fat
2,200 calories	24 grams saturated fat	73 grams total fat
2,500 calories	28 grams saturated fat	83 grams total fat
2,800 calories	31 grams saturated fat	93 grams total fat

If your LDL is over 100:

1,200 calories	8 grams saturated fat	33 grams total fat
1,600 calories	11 grams saturated fat	44 grams total fat
2,000 calories	16 grams saturated fat	55 grams total fat
2,200 calories	17 grams saturated fat	61 grams total fat
2,500 calories	19 grams saturated fat	69 grams total fat
2,800 calories	22 grams saturated fat	78 grams total fat

Are Some Cuts of Meat Less Fatty Than Others?

Absolutely, and they are outlined below.

Beef. Top round, eye of round, round steak, rump roast, sirloin tip, short loin, strip steak, lean and extra lean ground beef

Pork. Tenderloin, sirloin roast or chop, center cut loin chops

Lamb. Foreshank, leg roast, leg chop, loin chop

What's the Best Way To Cook To Reduce Fat?

Many options are available when it comes cooking healthy. If you are careful to not add butter or fat-laden sauces, keeping your heart in great shape is easy. You can bake, broil, grill, microwave, poach, roast, steam, or lightly stir-fry or sauté in cooking spray, a small amount of vegetable oil, or reduced sodium broth.

Chapter 7

◆ ◆ ❖ ◆ ◆ ❖ ◆ ◆ ❖ ◆ ◆ ❖ ◆ ◆ ❖ ◆ ◆ ❖ ◆ ◆

The Savvy Shopper

Let the Nutrition Facts Label
Guide You to Healthy Choices

Let's face it—food shopping can be frustrating. Shelves are packed with products stating, "low this" and "high that." Some even have special health claims. How do we sort through it all? Using the Nutrition Facts Panel on food labels will greatly simplify things as well as help maintain your sanity!

There are two parts to the Nutrition Facts Panel. The top part contains product specific information including serving size, calories, and specific nutrient amounts present in the food. This information varies from product to product. The second part is the footnote and it is found only on larger packages. The footnote provides general guidelines on recommended intakes of specific nutrients according to calorie intake.

Because the serving size noted on the package influences all of the nutrient amounts listed on the label, this is the first area that you'll want to lay your eyes on. Compare the serving size indicated to the amount that you actually eat. You can then accurately determine how much of a specific nutrient you are consuming. For example, if the serving size is ½ cup and you plan on eating one cup, then all the nutrient information listed must be doubled to determine the correct amount that you have ingested. If you consume only one-fourth cup, the information will need to be halved. See the sample nutrition facts panel below.

Nutrition Facts

Serving Size ½ cup (67g)
Servings Per Container 16
Amount Per Serving
Calories 100 Calories from Fat 0
% Daily Value
Total Fat 0g 0%
Saturated Fat 0g 0%
Cholesterol 0g 0%
Sodium 60mg 3%
Total Carbohydrate 22g 7%
Dietary Fiber 0g 0%
Sugars 15g
Protein 3g
Vitamin A 2%
Vitamin C* 0%
Calcium 45%
Iron* 0%
*Percent Daily Values are based on a 2,000 calorie diet.

Another useful tool present on the label is the Percent Daily Value (%DV). This makes it easy to note whether a food is a poor or rich source of a specific nutrient. Following the "5 to 20 rule" assists you in quickly assessing if the product contains small or large amounts of a particular nutrient. It also allows you to rapidly compare different foods for nutrient content. If the %DV is less than 5, the food is low in that nutrient. On the other hand, if the %DV is greater than 20, the item is an excellent source of the nutrient. With the %DV, there is no need to memorize the definitions of claims such as "light", "nonfat" or "low-fat." One glance at the %DV for total fat will clue you in on which item is higher or lower in fat. Just because a food is high in a non–heart-healthy nutrient (like saturated fat, cholesterol, or sodium), doesn't mean that you must give it up. Just choose foods lower in that nutrient the rest of the day in order to balance things out.

Percent Daily Values are based on the needs of a person consuming 2,000 calories per day. Even if your caloric intake is different from this, you can still use the information to quickly compare food products.

Another useful part of the food label is the ingredient list. It tells you what's in the food—including any added nutrients, fats, or sugars. Ingredients are listed by weight from most to least. If a product states "with real fruit juice added" and on the ingredient list you see that fruit juice is listed as the fourteenth ingredient, you know that very little juice is actually in the product.

Learn the Label Language

Prior to 1993 claims on label such as free, low, light, and high, were not regulated and were only marketing hype. This is true no longer. The Food and Drug Administration along with the U.S. Department of Agriculture's Food Safety and Inspection Service have set labeling regulations, reestablishing the credibility of claims on food labels. Heart-healthy products are often flagged with terms such as "low-fat," "low-sodium," and "low calorie." Regulated terms and their meanings are described below.

SODIUM	WHAT IT MEANS
Sodium free or salt free	Less than 5 milligrams per serving
Very low-sodium	35 milligrams or less per serving
low-sodium	140 milligrams or less per serving
low-sodium meal	140 milligrams or less per 3½ ounces (100 grams)
Reduced or less sodium	At least 25 percent less sodium than the regular version
Light in sodium	Half the sodium of the regular version
Unsalted or no salt added	No salt added to the product during processing

FATS	WHAT IT MEANS
Fat-free	Less than 0.5 grams per serving
Low saturated fat	1 gram or less per serving
Low-fat	3 grams or less per serving
Reduced fat	At least 25 percent less fat than the regular version
Light in fat	Half the fat of the regular version

CALORIES	WHAT IT MEANS
Calorie free	Less than 5 calories per serving
Low calorie	40 calories or less per serving
Reduced or less calories	At least 25 percent fewer calories than the regular version
Light or lite	Half the fat or a third of the calories of the regular version

Food Label Savvy

Take a moment to think about your financial budget. A budget consists of a variety of expenses including housing, travel, clothing, food, and health insurance. If you stick to a cost-saving plan using coupons for purchases, taking public transportation or finding bargain sales at the mall, you have money left over to spend on luxury items. In this case, the goal is to get the biggest bang for your buck (so you can take that summer vacation!) Similarly, a successful calorie-saving plan depends on eating nutrient dense foods. Nutrient density refers to foods that deliver the most nutrients at a low calorie level, *saving* you from putting on extra pounds. In order to stay within your "calorie budget," aim to limit your intake of empty-calorie foods and beverages such as soda, candy, or "fat-free" items loaded with sugar. The following criteria will help you select nutrient dense foods based on information on the Nutrition Facts Label.

The Heart-Healthy Shopper

Healthy eating starts in your kitchen. It is easy to prepare nutritious meals by stocking your refrigerator, cupboards and freezer with healthy foods and ingredients. Have a snack craving? Smear a teaspoon of all natural peanut butter on a fresh apple picked from your fruit bowl, or whip up a smoothie using yogurt and frozen berries from the freezer. Foods high in saturated fat (like Ben and Jerry's ice cream) are less likely to tempt you if they are reserved as an occasional treat to enjoy outside your home. Following a heart-healthy diet is a lifestyle change but it should still be an enjoyable experience. The following food shopping tips will help you become supermarket savvy.

Prepare a list. Decide what to buy before you are tempted by the foods in the store. Just because chips are on sale, does not mean you have to buy them! Foods (especially high-fat sugar-laden foods) are strategically placed on supermarket shelves to attract consumers, so remember to only shop from the list!

Shop on a full stomach. It is easy to buy impulsively when you are hungry. An innocent trip to the grocery store to buy a few essen-

---

Food Label Savvy: Criteria To Super Snack Choices!

* Always read the 1st ingredient on the food label. This will help you determine how wholesome a product really is. Ingredients are always listed in descending order.
* Always look at the serving size on the label. The nutrient facts are translated on a per serving basis.

#1 Good Source of fiber = > 2.5 gm/ serving

When you are food shopping, look for the following:
   Cereal and Bread: 3 grams or more / serving
   As an added bonus, try high fiber cereal and bread: 5 grams or more / serving

#2 Percentage of calories from fat = <30% calories from fat

Note: Ignore this rule when it comes to eating healthy fats such as flaxseed, fatty fish, olive/canola/peanut oil, butter substitutes, hummus, all natural peanut butter, almonds/sesame seeds/walnuts. These foods contain heart-healthy monounsaturated fats or omega fats.

#3 Low in saturated fat = Less than 1 gram saturated fat / serving

Refer to tables on pages 55 to 56 to figure out your ideal saturated fat intake per day.

#4 Sugar = less than 5 grams of sugar/ serving

Aim for a maximum of 30 to 50 grams of sugar per day (8 to 12 teaspoons)
   1 teaspoon sugar = 4 grams = ~16 calories. Try to minimize your intake of foods with added sugar (sweetened cereals, foods with high fructose corn syrup). Instead, eat foods with natural sugars that also contain abundant vitamins and minerals (whole fruits)

#5 % Daily value for vitamins and minerals = 10 to 19% = Good Source >19% = Excellent source

---

tials can become an eating excursion. The heart-healthy shopper EATS beforehand to prevent temptation by food items high in saturated fat.

Buy foods that require preparation. Foods that come prepackaged may also be highly processed (high in saturated fat, transfat, or sodium). Buying food that requires preparation will encourage you to think about heart-healthy meals!

For example, let's say you crave chicken tonight. Think about buying a whole chicken. If you choose the "preparation route," you can decide how much you want to eat, how to prepare it (removing the skin and baking it). The result: you saved yourself over 200 calories compared to buying a 3-piece fried chicken dinner.

Don't forget store brands. These are usually less expensive and just as tasty!

Buy cheaper cuts of meat. Try cuts such as round, loin, and flank. They have less fat.

Choose red meat, rather than pink. This rule applies to buying ground beef. Select lean ground beef that has a bright cherry red color rather than meat that appears pink. Pink is created by mixing red and white. In this case, white represents undesirable saturated fat.

Be aware of code names for sugar. Other names for sugar include high fructose corn syrup, maltose, dextrose, high fructose corn syrup, fruit juice concentrate, sucrose, honey, and maple syrup. These ingredients are usually found in refined carbohydrates and empty calorie foods.

Read labels. Ingredients are listed in descending order. Imagine this scenario: You pick up a bag of fruit snacks that claims to be a "good source of vitamin C." While this may be true, you notice that one of the first few ingredients reads high fructose corn syrup (another word for added sugar and therefore extra calories) You are better off going for the fresh fruit which contains natural sugars packed with a variety of nutrients.

Healthy Shopping Strategies

The foods you buy set the stage for eating. Having problem foods available in the house, office, car, briefcase, or pocket can invite trouble even if you vow to "eat only a little." Instead, if you have wholesome foods readily available, you will be more likely to eat heart-healthy.

Don't be fooled by spray vs. tubs. The facts:
1 Tbsp of tub butter = 90 calories, 10 grams fat

1 Tbsp of butter = 50 calories, 5 grams fat

The heart-healthy shopper chooses the spray. It's calorie-free, cholesterol free, fat-free, and sodium free. Once you get over the mental aspect of "spraying your food," it serves as a great way to save on extra calorie consumption. Use it on bread or spray on popcorn for extra flavor.

Don't be fooled by reduced fat peanut butter. The facts:

2 Tbsp of full fat peanut butter: 16 grams of fat, 200 calories

2 Tbsp of reduced fat peanut butter: 12 grams of fat, 200 calories

Peanut butter is calorie-dense. "Natural" peanut butter is good for your health because it contains unsaturated fat and protein. Reduced fat peanut butter has 25% less fat than original. Why does reduced fat have the same number of calories as full-fat peanut butter? When fat is taken out, another ingredient takes its place. In this case, heart-healthy fat has been replaced with fillers (maltodextrin) along with unhealthy partially hydrogenated oils (trans-fats!). The heart-healthy shopper chooses the regular peanut butter and limits portion size.

Don't be fooled by claims such as:

"Eat Special K™ for 2 meals each day and lose six pounds in two weeks."

The heart-healthy shopper does not buy it for these reasons:

The ingredients: rice, wheat gluten, sugar

Not the whole grain (it's refined and processed—just like white bread)

1 cup is the equivalent of eating 1 slice of white bread. Just because a diet is low calorie, does not automatically mean it's heart-healthy!

Don't be fooled by 2% milk. The facts:

Whole milk is 3% fat

2% milk isn't much better; only 2% fat, contains 5 grams fat per cup (too much saturated fat). It is not considered a low-fat food. A low-fat food must have less than 3 grams of fat per serving.

The heart-healthy shopper chooses skim milk or 1% milk. If you like the consistency of whole milk without all the fat, choose Skim Plus (provides more protein and calcium).

Don't be fooled by 85% lean meat. The facts are food products are often labeled by weight, such as 85% lean meat or 85% fat-free. These foods may be only 15% fat by weight, but can provide over 50% of their calories from fat (heart-healthy guideline states: choose foods with <30% calories from fat, <10% calories from saturated fat).

The heart-healthy shopper knows to evaluate foods based on grams of fat per serving, total calories, and calories from fat.

Don't be fooled by wheat bread. The facts are darker bread is not always "healthy with fiber." Wheat bread is not always "made from whole grains."

The heart-healthy shopper knows to choose whole grain bread, pitas, bagels, and crackers by looking at the FIRST ingredient on the label: 100% whole wheat or 100% whole grain. Be careful with bagels. Most are so big that calories can easily reach 500! Select mini bagels if you are trying to lose weight. (1 mini bagel = 15 grams of carbohydrate = 1 serving of starch). Choose other breads over croissants and focaccia.

Don't be fooled by 7, 9 Grain Bread. The facts are these breads are usually just white bread sprinkled with a few other grains (not enough to make it heart-healthy). The heart-healthy shopper only buys it if "whole wheat" or "whole grain" flour is listed as the first ingredient. Also, check out the food label for at least 3 grams of fiber or more per slice.

Don't be fooled by energy bars. The facts are some bars are no more than glorified candy bars. Most bars are calorie-dense with little or no fiber, and many are high in saturated fat.

The heart-healthy shopper does not rely on energy bars as a primary nutrition source. They may be useful before or during an endurance exercise. Try not to spend more than $1.00–$1.50 on a bar. (Power Bar™ or Gatorade™ Energy Bar). Read food labels carefully and choose bars with fiber, less than 5 grams of fat, less than 30% calories from fat (Cliff Bar).

The Produce Aisle

The heart-healthy shopper knows that every choice is a good one, packed with beneficial vitamins, minerals, and phytochemicals. Phytochemicals are non-nutrient compounds that have biological activity. Flavanoids, a large group of phytochemicals are powerful antioxidants that may help to protect LDL from oxidation and reduce blood platelet stickiness. Keep in mind that the more color the fruit or vegetable has, the more nutrients. Some of the best fruit choices include: guava, watermelon, kiwifruit, papaya, cantaloupe, orange, strawberries, apricots, peaches, blackberries, raspberries, tangerine, mango, honeydew melon, and starfruit, among others.

The Dairy Case

The heart-healthy shopper knows to choose skim or 1% milk. Parmesan cheese goes a long way. Sprinkle on salad, veggies, and potatoes instead of full fat cheeses. Low-fat shredded cheeses are quick, good choices. Polly-O fat-free/low-fat string cheese is also a good snack. Make sure to choose low-fat and fat-free cheeses and save up to 10 grams of fat per ounce.

Yogurt is nutritious. One cup of yogurt can actually contain up to 400 mg of calcium (25% of your daily needs!) Choose fat-free, low-fat and "light" yogurt for fat and calorie savers. Try to find yogurts that contain active cultures. Active cultures are good for lactose intolerant people because they digest lactose for you.

The Heart-Healthy Shopper is NOT fooled by:

* *Cheez-Whiz™- it's processed and 2 Tbsp provide a whopping 200 calories and 9 grams of fat!*

* *Jell-O™ Brand, Colombo, and Light n Lively™ brands of yogurt contain less calcium.*

* *Snackwell's Brand™ fat-free yogurt doesn't contain active cultures and has a lot of added sugar, (thus extra calories and less calcium ounce for ounce).*

* *Coffee yogurt contains caffeine—which is not listed on the food label. Exceptions to the rule include Stonyfield Farm™ Nonfat Cappuccino and Dannon Light™ Cappuccino—they contain no caffeine.*

The heart-healthy shopper chooses egg scramblers—they're fat and cholesterol free! Two eggs whites can be substituted for one whole egg in a recipe.

Canned Goods: Soups and Sauces

The heart-healthy shopper pays attention to fat and sodium on food labels.

You should skip Campbells's traditional red and white label soups as well as Ramen Noodles and Cup O'Noodles™ soup which are fat-laden. A better choice for soups are bean, lentil, and split pea soups.

For pasta sauces, make sure you choose "skinny" pasta sauces. The best choice is fat-free sauce with no sodium added. Canned is fine, and you can add your own spices to Delmonte's or Hunts™ "no salt added" tomato sauce. You can also opt for a sauce with less than 3 grams of fat (ideally from heart-healthy olive oil) and 500 mg of sodium per ½ cup serving. Classico™ Fire Roasted Tomato and Garlic, Healthy Choice™ Varieties, and Five Brothers™ Oven Roasted Garlic and Onion are a few that meet this criteria. Many other brands pack up to 10 grams of fat and 1,000 mg of sodium per serving!

You should read ingredients and calories listed on tomato sauce- choose sauces with less than 100 calories per cup (Ragu™ Light, many Healthy Choice™ varieties, Hunts™, Dole™). Many sauces have added oils and meats (which gives you no option to choose lean meat) and really increases calories.

Frozen Food Aisle

The heart-healthy shopper knows that frozen dinners should have no more than 10 grams of fat, at least 3 grams of fiber, and less than 800 mg of sodium.
Good Choices:

* *Gardenburgers™ (Fire Roasted Vegetable, Sundried Tomato, etc.)—low-fat or fat-free. The same size "lean" ground beef burger contains 13 grams of fat.*
* *Green Giant™ ground soy crumbles can be used to replace the meat in sloppy joes and in spaghetti sauces.*
* *Yves™ wieners and Lightlife™ smart dogs.*
* *Morningstar Farms™ sausage patties or links*

* *Healthy Choice™, Smart Ones™, and Lean Cuisine™ Meals are fairly healthy but you may need to add a lot of fresh veggies if you don't want to finish your meal and still feel hungry.*

* *Better choices for pizza include Tombstone™ Light Vegetable Pizza, Wolfgang Puck's™ Fat-Free Cheeseless Grilled Vegetable or Mushroom and Spinach Pizza, Healthy Choice™ French Bread Pizza, Weight Watchers™, or Lean Cuisine™ French Bread Pizza.*

* *Cascadian Farms meals contain only about 4 grams of fat and 470 mg sodium.*

The heart-healthy shopper skips frozen food items such as pockets and pot pies. Pizzas made by Stouffer's™, Pappalo's™, Red Baron™, and Tony's are also on the reject list. Don't be fooled by hash browns-most are advertised as "fat-free". Those claims on their packages are no lies... until you follow the recommended cooking method, which will make it 8 to 29 grams of fat per serving!

Great picks for frozen desserts include Fat Free Edy's™ frozen yogurt—it tastes great and some flavors actually have 900 mg of calcium per cup, equivalent to the amount of calcium in 3 cups of milk. Other good choices include Fat Free Bryers, Fat Free Haagen-Dazs™, Healthy Choice™ Low Fat, fudge pops, and most sorbets.

Non-fat Reddi-Whip™, chocolate lite syrup, and frozen fruits are highly suggested, as well as fruit pops made with Splenda—great for diabetics as a sugar substitute!

The heart-healthy shopper skips Haagen-Dazs™, Ben and Jerry's™ and most other premium brands which have 40 grams fat/cup. If it's sitting in your freezer, it will eventually be eaten!

Cereal Aisle

Choose whole grain cereals. Great picks include cereals with at least 3 grams of fiber per serving (Kashi™, bran cereals). Fantastic brand instant oatmeal is quick, easy, and healthy.

Be careful with granola. Granola cereal may be made with whole grains but packs in a lot of fat. Choose a low-fat option. Beware of sugar cereals strategically placed at kids eye level. The healthiest way to cut down on sugar is to buy an unsweetened whole grain cereal like Wheatena™, oatmeal, oat bran, or Shredded Wheat and add your own fruit and low-fat milk.

If a cereal bar says it's healthy doesn't mean it is a good breakfast choice. Examples include Entenmann's™ Multi-Grain Real Apple Raisin bar, which boasts "made with real apples." The package doesn't mention that they're mostly white flour and sugar. If you want one of those "real apples" on the label, you would have to eat roughly 70 bars to get it!

Condiment Aisle

When purchasing mayonnaise, select "light" or "free" products. Remember that mustard is calorie and fat-free. Be cautious if you have high blood pressure because the sodium adds up quickly in most condiments. Try low-sodium versions of soy sauce and teriyaki sauces. 2 Tbsp of regular soy sauce equals 2424 mg of sodium which exceeds your daily need of sodium!

Choose nonfat or low-fat versions of salad dressing. Examples include balsamic vinegar, lemon, salsa. Salad dressing can be a BIG contributor of fat in your diet—2 Tbsp of regular dressing can pile on as many as 300 calories and 10 to 25 grams of fat! All natural peanut butters like Smucker's™ All Natural are a better choice than processed brands.

Meat and Poultry Aisle

Choose turkey and chicken breast without skin. For example, select Boar's Head™ at the deli counter. Round and loin cuts of beef are the healthiest for your heart. When selecting pork, your best bet is loin, pork chop sirloin roast, trimmed. This choice will save you 24 grams of fat compared to spareribs, untrimmed.

Choose fish–any type of fish!! Just don't fry. The fattier fish such as salmon, tuna, and mackerel provide beneficial omega-3 fatty acids! Buy canned tuna and salmon in water, not in oil.

When selecting lunch meats, switch from high fat to lower fat hot dogs, sausage, ham, bacon, or bologna. These processed meats are a big contributor of fat in the average American's diet. Look for lower sodium varieties. Low-fat or fat-free bologna and hot dogs made by Healthy Choice™, Oscar Mayer™, and Hormel™ are good choices. Try Lois Rich™ or Oscar Mayer™ turkey bacon or low-fat ham. Try low-fat sausage made by Healthy Choice™ and others. Skip over Oscar Mayer™ "Lunchables." Two-thirds of the calories come from fats and sugars.

Butter and Margarine

Butter is the culprit for saturated fat, whereas margarine is the culprit for trans-fat. Your best bet is going with low calorie, fat-free options. Choose I Can't Believe It's Not Butter Spray, Butter Buds™, Molly McButter™ (check out all the different varieties including cheese sprinkles), and Mrs. Dash™ varieties.

For sticks, choose Fleischmanns trans-free spread or Promise. You may also want to try Smart Beat Super Light, Fleischmann's™ Lower Fat, Promise Ultra 70% Less Fat. These varieties all taste great, and have 2 to 5 grams of fat per tablespoon. They also have no more than 1 gram of the "bad" fat. However, keep in mind they still have many calories.

Microwave popcorn

Popcorn can be a nutritious snack and a good source of fiber if you choose healthy varieties. The good news is that 3 cups of popcorn contain only 50 to 70 calories, 1 to 3 grams of fat. Best picks include Healthy Choice™, Orville Redenbacher's™ Smart Pop! / Natural Light, and Low-fat Newman's Own™ Light.

The bad news is that 3 cups of popcorn can also contain 110-150 calories, 7 to 12 grams of fat if you go with high fat, butter varieties. The heart-healthy shopper skips Redeb-Budders, Orville Redenbacher's™ Butter, Pop-Secret™ Butter, Natural or Real Butter Popcorn. Remember, food labels with the words "hydrogenated vegetable fat," or vegetable shortening mean that they contain undesirable trans-fats!

Quickie meals

By stocking up on good nutrition, you can pull together a no-cook meal or quickly prepare a hot dinner. The key is to stock basic foods that don't spoil easily: Consider these "quickie meals":

* *Whole grain English muffin pizza*
* *Stone wheat crackers, peanut butter, low-fat/skim milk*
* *Lentil soup with extra broccoli, leftover pasta, a sprinkling of Parmesan*
* *Tuna on whole wheat bread with salad (spinach, lettuce, tomato, carrots, beans, peppers... with 1 to 2 Tbsp low-fat dressing)*
* *Bran cereal with banana and strawberries*

CUPBOARD	REFRIGERATOR	FREEZER
Whole wheat spaghetti	Low-fat cheese	English muffins
Rice	Grated parmesan	Pita bread (whole wheat)
Potatoes	Low-fat cottage cheese	Multigrain bread
Wheat crackers	Low-fat yogurt	Broccoli
Spaghetti sauce	Low-fat milk/skim plus	Spinach
Pretzels	Egg beaters	Winter squash
Tuna	Oranges	Spinach
Canned salmon	Bananas	Skinless and boneless
Kidney beans	Carrots, cucumbers, peppers	chicken breast
Peanut butter	Whole wheat tortilla	Extra-lean hamburger
High-fiber cereal	Tofu	Frozen fruit
Oatmeal	Apples, peaches, pears	Turkey breast
Raisins		Vegetable burgers

Freezing does not destroy a food's nutritional value. Frozen veggies also contain less salt than canned! Buy foods in season, because they are less expensive. Wilted, overripe, or bruised fruits and veggies indicate nutrient losses. Choose these foods carefully from the supermarket.

Recipe for Heart-Healthy Dip

NUTRITIONAL FACTS	
CALORIES:	217.10 KCALS
PROTEIN:	10.53G
CARBS:	18.55G
TOTAL FAT:	11.61G
SAT FAT:	4.53G
CHOLESTEROL:	13.29MG
SODIUM:	393.57MG
FIBER:	2.29G
CALCIUM:	50.78MG
POTASSIUM	169.81MG
YIELD:	8 SERVINGS
SERVING SIZE: 4 WHOLE WHEAT CRACKERS, ¼ CUP OF DIP	

1 8 oz package low-fat Philadelphia cream cheese, softened
1 can salsa (< 200 mg sodium per serving on the food label or refer to salsa recipe) diced vegetables (tomatoes, onions, scallions, peppers, lettuce, carrots)
1 cup fat-free shredded cheddar cheese olives to garnish
Kavli whole-grain crackers or carrot sticks

---

1. Combine the cream cheese and salsa in a bowl. Mix well.
2. Spoon mixture onto serving platter. Layer vegetables on top.
3. Sprinkle cheese and garnish with a small ring of olives.
4. Serve with Kavli whole-grain crackers or carrot sticks.

This recipe is a creative way to boost your vegetable intake. It is a healthier alternative to a prepared dip loaded with calories and saturated fat. Make sure to select a fat-free shredded cheese that provides at least 10% of the Daily Value for calcium.

Take Home Message

Eliminating too much is not the answer... Eating healthy is about adding tasty foods to your diet that will deliver nutrients, provide sustained energy, and support lifelong health. Happy shopping!

Chapter 8

◆ ◆ ❖ ◆ ◆ ❖ ◆ ◆ ❖ ◆ ◆ ❖ ◆ ◆ ❖ ◆ ◆ ❖ ◆ ◆

Soups

When the air dons a chill, nothing warms us up better than a delicious bowl of soup! The old expression "all of nature's goodness in one spoon" is pretty accurate—soup is satisfying, easy to prepare and loaded with a variety of nutrients. It is a great dish to serve company because it can simmer an extra hour or two if necessary. Soups can also be frozen and reheated with ease. The soup recipes in this chapter contain relatively few calories, making them perfect for the weight conscious. Most are a good source of fiber and they are much lower in sodium than their canned counterparts. They taste better too!

Most soups call for an abundance of vegetables. What points should you consider when purchasing these? Freshness and quality! Characteristics of freshness include brightness and crispness. Avoid buying vegetables with decay, for rapid deterioration will still occur even after you've trimmed off the decayed area. Most fresh vegetables can be stored for two to five days. Root vegetables can be stored from one to several weeks.

Onions, celery, carrots, and cabbage are used frequently in soup recipes. When choosing onions, look for hard, firm, dry onions with small necks. Onions that have wet or soft necks are affected by decay, or have been picked too early. Also avoid purchasing those with thick, hollow, woody centers in the neck, those with fresh sprouts, and those containing green sunburn spots or other blemishes. Glossy, light to medium green celery stalks that feel solid and rigid, combined with non-wilted green leaflets are the best. Celery branch centers with brown or black discoloration, celery that is wilted, or celery showing signs of insect damage should not be purchased. Choose carrots that are firm, colorful, smooth, and well formed. Wilted carrots and those with green sunspots across the top should be avoided. Cabbage with dried, discolored, or decayed outer leaves that easily separate from the base of the head is not fresh. Instead, choose heavy, firm heads that have good green or red color and are free from blemishes. Remember, high quality ingredients result in a superior product!

Bean and Macaroni Soup

2 cans (16 oz each) great northern beans
1 Tbsp olive oil
½ lb fresh mushrooms, sliced
2 cups carrots, sliced
1 cup onion, coarsely chopped
1 cup celery, coarsely chopped
1 clove garlic, minced
3 cups tomatoes, fresh, peeled, cut up
  (or 1½ lb canned, whole, cut up)★
1 tsp dried sage
1 tsp dried thyme
½ tsp dried oregano
  to taste black pepper, freshly ground
1 bay leaf, crumbled
4 cups elbow macaroni, cooked

NUTRITIONAL FACTS	
CALORIES:	158
TOTAL FAT: 1 G	
SATURATED FAT:	LESS THAN 1 G
CHOLESTEROL:	0 MG
SODIUM:	154 MG
TOTAL FIBER:	5 MG
PROTEIN:	8 MG
CARBOHYDRATES:	29 G
POTASSIUM:	524 MG
YIELD:	16 SERVINGS
SERVING SIZE:	1 CUP

★ If using canned tomatoes, sodium content will be higher. Try "no salt added" canned tomatoes to keep sodium lower.

1. Drain beans and reserve liquid. Rinse beans.
2. Heat oil in 6-quart kettle. Add mushrooms, onion, carrots, celery, and garlic and sauté for 5 minutes.
3. Add tomatoes, sage, thyme, oregano, pepper, and bay leaf. Cover and cook over medium heat for 20 minutes.
4. Cook macaroni according to directions on package, using unsalted water. Drain when cooked. Do not overcook.
5. Combine reserved bean liquid with water to make 4 cups.
6. Add liquid, beans, and cooked macaroni to vegetable mixture.
7. Bring to a boil. Cover and simmer until soup is thoroughly heated. Stir occasionally.

This satisfying dish is virtually fat-free—it uses just 1 Tbsp of oil for 16 servings.

Cannery Row Soup

2 Tbsp olive oil
3 carrots, cut in thin strips
2 cups celery, sliced
½ cup onion, chopped
¼ cup green peppers, chopped
1 clove garlic, minced
1 can (28 oz) whole tomatoes, cut up,
   with liquid
1 cup clam juice
¼ tsp dried thyme, crushed
¼ tsp dried basil, crushed
⅛ tsp black pepper
2 lb varied fish fillets (such as haddock, perch, flounder, cod, sole), cut
   into 1-inch cubes
¼ cup fresh parsley, minced

NUTRITIONAL FACTS	
CALORIES:	170
TOTAL FAT:	5 G
SATURATED FAT:	LESS THAN 1 G
CHOLESTEROL:	56 MG
SODIUM:	380 MG
TOTAL FIBER:	3 G
PROTEIN:	22 G
CARBOHYDRATES:	9 G
POTASSIUM:	710 MG
YIELD:	8 SERVINGS
SERVING SIZE:	1 CUP

1. Heat oil in large saucepan. Sauté garlic, carrots, celery, onion, and green pepper in oil for 3 minutes.
2. Add remaining ingredients, except for parsley and fish. Cover and simmer for 10 to 15 minutes or until vegetables are fork tender.
3. Add fish and parsley. Simmer covered for 5 to 10 minutes more or until fish flakes easily and is opaque. Serve hot.

Fish and clam juice give this soup a hearty taste of the sea.

Corn Chowder

1 Tbsp vegetable oil
2 Tbsp celery, finely diced
2 Tbsp onion, finely diced
2 Tbsp green pepper, finely diced
1 package (10 oz) frozen whole kernel corn
1 cup raw potatoes, peeled, diced in ½-inch pieces
¼ tsp salt
   to taste black pepper
¼ tsp paprika
2 cups low-fat or skim milk
2 Tbsp flour
2 Tbsp fresh parsley, chopped

NUTRITIONAL FACTS	
CALORIES:	186
TOTAL FAT:	5 G
SATURATED FAT:	1 G
CHOLESTEROL:	5 MG
SODIUM:	205 MG
TOTAL FIBER:	4 G
PROTEIN:	7 G
CARBOHYDRATES:	31 G
POTASSIUM:	455 MG
YIELD:	4 SERVINGS
SERVING SIZE:	1 CUP

1. Heat oil in medium saucepan. Add celery, onion, and green pepper, and sauté for 2 minutes.

2. Add corn, potatoes, 1 cup of water, salt, pepper, and paprika. Bring to a boil, then reduce heat to medium. Cook covered for about 10 minutes or until potatoes are tender.

3. Place ½ cup of milk in a jar with tight fitting lid. Add flour and shake vigorously.

4. Gradually add milk-flour mixture to cooked vegetables. Then add remaining milk.

5. Cook, stirring constantly, until mixture comes to a boil and thickens. Serve garnished with chopped, fresh parsley.

Here's a creamy chowder without the cream—or fat.

Curtido (Cabbage) Salvadoreño

1 medium head of cabbage, chopped
2 small carrots, grated
1 small onion, sliced
½ cup vinegar
1 tsp olive oil
1 tsp salt
1 tsp brown sugar
½ tsp dried red pepper (optional)
½ tsp oregano

NUTRITIONAL FACTS

CALORIES:	41
TOTAL FAT:	1 G
SATURATED FAT:	LESS THAN 1 G
CHOLESTEROL:	0 MG
SODIUM:	293 MG
TOTAL FIBER:	2 G
PROTEIN:	2 G
CARBOHYDRATES:	7 G
POTASSIUM:	325 MG
YIELD:	8 SERVINGS
SERVING SIZE:	1 CUP

1. Blanch cabbage with boiling water for 1 minute. Discard water.
2. Place cabbage in a large bowl and add grated carrots, sliced onion, vinegar, olive oil, salt, brown sugar, pepper, oregano, and ½ cup water.
3. Place in refrigerator for at least 2 hours before serving.

Surprise your taste buds with this flavorful dish—esta terrifica!
Try this dish with Pupusas Revueltas.

Gazpacho

3 medium tomatoes, peeled, chopped
2 green onions, sliced
2 cups low-sodium vegetable juice cocktail
1 clove garlic, minced
½ cup cucumber, seeded, chopped
½ cup green pepper, chopped
1 Tbsp lemon juice
½ tsp basil, dried
¼ tsp hot pepper sauce

1. In large mixing bowl, combine all the ingredients.
2. Cover and chill in the refrigerator for several hours.

This chilled tomato soup is a classic—and chock full of healthy garden-fresh vegetables.

NUTRITIONAL FACTS	
CALORIES:	52
TOTAL FAT:	LESS THAN 1 G
SATURATED FAT:	LESS THAN 1 G
CHOLESTEROL:	0 MG
SODIUM:	41 MG
TOTAL FIBER:	2 G
PROTEIN:	2 G
CARBOHYDRATES:	12 G
POTASSIUM:	514 MG
YIELD:	4 SERVINGS
SERVING SIZE:	1¼ CUPS

Homemade Turkey Soup

6 lb turkey breast with bones
(with at least 2 cups meat)

2 medium onions

3 stalks celery

1 tsp dried thyme

1 tsp dried basil

½ tsp dried rosemary

½ tsp dried sage

½ tsp dried marjoram

½ tsp dried tarragon

½ tsp salt

to taste black pepper

½ lb Italian pastina or pasta

NUTRITIONAL FACTS	
CALORIES:	201
TOTAL FAT:	2 G
SATURATED FAT:	1 G
CHOLESTEROL:	101 MG
SODIUM:	141 MG
TOTAL FIBER:	1 G
PROTEIN:	33 G
CARBOHYDRATES:	11 G
POTASSIUM:	344 MG
YIELD:	16 SERVINGS
(ABOUT 4 QUARTS OF SOUP)	
SERVING SIZE:	1 CUP

1. Place the turkey breast in large 6-quart pot. Cover with water until at least three quarters full.
2. Peel the onions, cut into large pieces, and add to the pot. Wash the celery stalks, slice, and add to pot.
3. Simmer covered for about 2½ hours.
4. Remove carcass from pot. Divide soup into smaller, shallower containers for quick cooling in refrigerator.
5. After cooling, skim off fat.
6. While soup cools, remove remaining meat from turkey carcass. Cut into pieces.
7. Add turkey meat to skimmed soup, along with herbs and spices.
8. Bring to boil and add pastina. Continue cooking on a low boil for about 20 minutes or until pastina is done. Serve at once or refrigerate for later reheating.

This popular soup uses a "quick cool down" that lets you skim the fat right off the top—making it even healthier.

Meatball Soup

1 small onion, chopped

½ cup green pepper, chopped

1 tsp mint

1 Tbsp annato (also called achiote), optional, for coloring

1 bay leaf

½ lb ground chicken

½ lb ground lean beef

2 small tomatoes, chopped

2 cloves garlic, minced

4 Tbsp instant corn flour

½ tsp oregano

½ tsp black pepper

½ tsp salt

2 medium carrots, chopped

2 celery stalks, chopped

2 cups cabbage, chopped

1 medium chayote, chopped (added zucchini can be used instead)

1 package (10 oz) frozen corn

2 medium zucchini, chopped

½ cup cilantro, minced

NUTRITIONAL FACTS	
CALORIES:	161
TOTAL FAT:	4 G
SATURATED FAT:	1 G
CHOLESTEROL:	31 MG
SODIUM:	193 MG
TOTAL FIBER:	4 G
PROTEIN:	13 G
CARBOHYDRATES:	17 G
POTASSIUM:	461 MG
YIELD:	8 SERVINGS
SERVING SIZE:	1¼ CUPS

1. In large pot, combine 10 cups of water, half of the onion, green pepper, annato, bay leaf, and ½ teaspoon of mint. Bring to a boil.
2. In bowl, combine chicken, beef, other half of onion, tomato, garlic, corn flour, oregano, pepper, and salt. Mix well. Form 1-inch meatballs. Place meatballs in boiling water and lower the heat. Cook over low heat for 30 to 45 minutes.
3. Add carrots, celery, cabbage, and chayote. Cook over low heat for 25 minutes. Add corn and zucchini. Cook for another 5 minutes. Garnish with cilantro and the rest of the mint.

This soup beefs up the health by using chicken with lean beef to lower the fat.

Mexican Pozole

1 Tbsp olive oil

2 lb lean beef, cubed*

1 large onion, chopped

1 clove garlic, finely chopped

¼ cup cilantro

¼ tsp salt

⅛ tsp pepper

1 can (15 oz) stewed tomatoes

2 oz tomato paste

1 can (1 lb 13 oz) hominy

NUTRITIONAL FACTS	
CALORIES:	253
TOTAL FAT:	10 G
SATURATED FAT:	3 G
CHOLESTEROL:	52 MG
SODIUM:	425 MG
TOTAL FIBER:	4 G
PROTEIN:	22 G
CARBOHYDRATES:	19 G
POTASSIUM:	485 MG
YIELD:	10 SERVINGS
SERVING SIZE:	1 CUP

* Skinless, boneless chicken breasts can be used instead of beef cubes.

1. In large pot, heat oil, then sauté beef.

2. Add onion, garlic, cilantro, salt, pepper, and enough water to cover meat. Cover pot and cook over low heat until meat is tender.

3. Add tomatoes and tomato paste. Continue cooking for about 20 minutes.

4. Add hominy and continue cooking over low heat for another 15 minutes, stirring occasionally. If too thick, add more water for desired consistency.

Try a change of taste with this hearty Mexican soup.

Minestrone Soup

¼ cup olive oil

1½ cups celery with leaves, coarsely chopped

1⅓ cups onion, coarsely chopped

1 clove garlic, minced (or ⅛ tsp powder)

1 can (1 lb) tomatoes, cut up

1 can (6 oz) tomato paste

4¾ cups cabbage, shredded

1 cup canned red kidney beans, drained, rinsed

1 cup carrots, sliced, fresh or frozen

1½ cups frozen peas

1½ cups fresh green beans

1 Tbsp fresh parsley, chopped

dash hot sauce

2 cups spaghetti, uncooked, broken

NUTRITIONAL FACTS	
CALORIES:	112
TOTAL FAT:	4 G
SATURATED FAT:	0 G
CHOLESTEROL:	0 MG
SODIUM:	202 MG
TOTAL FIBER:	4 G
PROTEIN:	4 G
CARBOHYDRATES:	17 G
POTASSIUM:	393 MG
YIELD:	16 SERVINGS
SERVING SIZE:	1 CUP

1. Heat oil in 4-quart saucepan. Add celery, onion, and garlic, and sauté for about 5 minutes.

2. Add tomato, tomato paste, cabbage, kidney beans, carrots, peas, green beans, parsley, hot sauce, and 11 cups of water. Stir until ingredients are well mixed.

3. Bring to a boil and reduce heat. Cover and simmer for about 45 minutes or until vegetables are tender.

4. Add uncooked spaghetti and simmer for only 2 to 3 minutes.

This cholesterol-free version of the classic Italian soup is brimming with fiber-rich beans, peas, and carrots.

Pupusas Revueltas

1 lb chicken breast, ground
1 Tbsp vegetable oil
½ small onion, finely diced
1 clove garlic, minced
1 medium green pepper, seeded, minced
1 small tomato, finely chopped
½ lb low-fat mozzarella cheese, grated
5 cups instant corn flour (masa harina)

NUTRITIONAL FACTS	
CALORIES:	290
TOTAL FAT:	7 G
SATURATED FAT:	3 G
CHOLESTEROL:	33 MG
SODIUM:	223 MG
TOTAL FIBER:	5 G
PROTEIN:	14 G
CARBOHYDRATES:	38 G
POTASSIUM:	272 MG
YIELD:	12 SERVINGS
SERVING SIZE:	2 PUPUSAS

1. In nonstick skillet, sauté chicken in oil over low heat until it turns white. Stir chicken constantly to keep it from sticking.
2. Add onion, garlic, green pepper, and tomato. Cook chicken mixture through. Remove skillet from stove and let mixture cool in refrigerator.
3. Meanwhile, place flour in large mixing bowl and stir in enough water to make stiff, tortilla-like dough.
4. When chicken mixture has cooled, mix in cheese.
5. Divide dough into 24 portions. With your hands, roll dough into balls and flatten each into ½ inch thick circle. Put spoonful of chicken mixture in middle of each circle of dough and bring edges to center. Flatten ball of dough again until it is ½ inch thick.
6. In very hot iron skillet, cook pupusas on each side until golden brown. Serve hot.

Try this dish with Curtido Salvadoreño. Ground chicken and low-fat cheese help keep down the fat and calories in this tasty dish.

Rockport Fish Chowder

2 Tbsp vegetable oil
½ cup celery, coarsely chopped
¼ cup onion, coarsely chopped
2 cups bottled clam juice
2 cups potatoes, raw, peeled, cubed
1 cup carrots, sliced
½ tsp paprika
¼ tsp thyme
8 whole peppercorns
1 bay leaf
1 lb fresh or frozen (and thawed) cod or
   haddock fillets, cut into ¾–inch cubes
3 cups low-fat milk
¼ cup flour
1 Tbsp fresh parsley, chopped

NUTRITIONAL FACTS	
CALORIES:	186
TOTAL FAT:	6 G
SATURATED FAT:	1 G
CHOLESTEROL:	34 MG
SODIUM:	302 MG
TOTAL FIBER:	2 G
PROTEIN:	15 G
CARBOHYDRATES:	18 G
POTASSIUM:	602 MG
YIELD:	8 SERVINGS
SERVING SIZE:	1 CUP

1. Heat oil in large saucepan. Add celery and onion, and sauté for about 3 minutes.

2. Add clam broth, potatoes, carrots, paprika, and thyme. Wrap peppercorns and bay leaf in cheese cloth. Add to pot. Bring to boil, reduce heat, and simmer for 15 minutes, then add fish and simmer for an added 15 minutes, or until fish flakes easily and is opaque.

3. Remove fish and vegetables. Break fish into chunks. Bring broth to boil and continue boiling until volume is reduced to 1 cup. Remove bay leaf and peppercorns.

4. Shake flour and ½ cup low-fat milk in container with tight-fitting lid until smooth. Add to broth in saucepan, along with remaining milk. Cook over medium heat, stirring constantly, until mixture boils and is thickened.

5. Return vegetables and fish chunks to stock and heat thoroughly. Serve hot, sprinkled with chopped parsley.

Serve this chowder as an appetizer or meal in itself—and eat like an admiral on a health cruise.

Chapter 9

♦ ♦ ❖ ♦ ♦ ❖ ♦ ♦ ❖ ♦ ♦ ❖ ♦ ♦ ❖ ♦ ♦ ❖ ♦ ♦

Meats (Beef, Pork, Veal, and Lamb)

Yes, you can enjoy meat while retaining a heart-healthy diet. The recipes comprising this chapter show you how. Besides being an outstanding source of protein, meat (beef, pork, veal, and lamb) contains significant amounts of the vitamins B6, B12, panthothenic acid, and phosphorus. It is also packed with the minerals iron and zinc. Many of these mentioned vitamins assist in energy production as well as DNA, nerve, and red blood cell formation. Iron is part of hemoglobin, a molecule that carries oxygen to the cells. Without zinc, our wounds would not be able to heal.

Because many meats are high in cholesterol and saturated fat, care must be taken to purchase the leanest cuts available. Choose USDA Choice or Select grades rather than USDA prime which has a higher fat content. Look for meat that has the least amount of visible fat, both around the edges and marbled through it. For ground beef, check the label and purchase only those with a fat content of 10 percent or lower. Select meats that are red or pink in color. This is a sign of freshness. Vacuum-packed meats may look a little purple in color, this is okay, it's just due to lack of exposure to air.

Meat should remain in its original store packaging until you are ready to use it and it must be kept cold. If you aren't planning to cook the meat within three days of purchase, freeze it. Ground meat needs to be frozen if it's not prepared within two days. Whole cuts of meat can be frozen for one year and ground meats for nearly four months. Be sure to thaw meat in the refrigerator thoroughly prior to cooking. If time is short, you can defrost it in the microwave or run the sealed package under cold water. Be sure to avoid thawing meat at room temperature because it promotes the growth of bacteria, leading to food poisoning.

Bavarian Beef

1¼ lb lean beef stew meat, trimmed of fat, cut
    in 1-inch pieces
1 Tbsp vegetable oil
1 large onion, thinly sliced
¾ tsp caraway seeds
½ tsp salt
⅛ tsp black pepper
1 bay leaf
¼ cup white vinegar
1 Tbsp sugar
½ small head red cabbage, cut into 4 wedges
¼ cup gingersnaps, crushed

NUTRITIONAL FACTS	
CALORIES:	218
TOTAL FAT:	7 G
SATURATED FAT:	2 G
CHOLESTEROL:	60 MG
SODIUM:	323 MG
TOTAL FIBER:	2 G
PROTEIN:	24 G
CARBOHYDRATES:	14 G
POTASSIUM:	509 MG
YIELD:	5 SERVINGS
SERVING SIZE:	5 OZ

1. Brown meat in oil in heavy skillet. Remove meat and sauté onion in remaining oil until golden. Return meat to skillet. Add 1½ cup water, caraway seeds, salt, pepper, and bay leaf. Bring to a boil. Reduce heat, cover, and simmer for 1¼ hours.
2. Add vinegar and sugar, and stir. Place cabbage on top of meat. Cover and simmer for 45 minutes.
3. Remove meat and cabbage, arrange on platter, and keep warm.
4. Strain drippings from skillet and skim off fat. Add enough water to drippings to yield 1 cup of liquid.
5. Return to skillet with crushed gingersnaps. Cook and stir until thickened and mixture boils. Pour over meat and vegetables, and serve.

This classic German stew is made with lean, trimmed beef stew meat and cabbage.

Beef and Bean Chili

2 lb lean beef stew meat, trimmed of fat,
  cut in 1-inch cubes
3 Tbsp vegetable oil
1 large onion, finely chopped
2 tsp garlic, minced
1 Tbsp flour
2 lb (or 3 cup) tomatoes, chopped
2 cups canned kidney beans★
1 green pepper, chopped
1 Tbsp oregano
2 tsp chili powder
1 tsp cumin

NUTRITIONAL FACTS	
CALORIES:	284
TOTAL FAT:	10 G
SATURATED FAT:	2 G
CHOLESTEROL:	76 MG
SODIUM:	162 MG
TOTAL FIBER:	4 G
PROTEIN:	33 G
CARBOHYDRATES:	16 G
POTASSIUM:	769 MG
YIELD:	9 SERVINGS
SERVING SIZE:	8 OZ

★ To cut back on sodium, try using "no salt added" canned kidney beans or beans prepared at home without salt.

1. Brown meat in large skillet with half of the vegetable oil. Add 2 cups of water. Simmer covered for 1 hour until meat is tender.
2. Heat remaining vegetable oil in a second skillet. Add onion and garlic, and cook over low heat until onion is softened. Add flour and cook for 2 minutes.
3. Add the garlic and onion mixture to the cooked meat. Then add remaining ingredients to meat mixture. Simmer for ½ hour.

Here's a lower fat chili that lost none of its heat.

Beef Stroganoff

1 lb lean beef (top round), cubed
2 tsp vegetable oil
¾ Tbsp onion, finely chopped
1 lb mushrooms, sliced
½ tsp dried basil
¼ tsp salt
¼ tsp nutmeg
  to taste pepper
1 cup plain low-fat yogurt
¼ cup white wine
6 cups macaroni, cooked in unsalted water

NUTRITIONAL FACTS	
CALORIES:	499
TOTAL FAT:	10 G
SATURATED FAT:	3 G
CHOLESTEROL:	80 MG
SODIUM:	200 MG
TOTAL FIBER:	4 G
PROTEIN:	41 G
CARBOHYDRATES:	58 G
POTASSIUM:	891 MG
YIELD:	5 SERVINGS
SERVING SIZE:	6 OZ

1. Cut beef into 1-inch cubes.
2. Heat 1 teaspoon oil in nonstick skillet. Sauté onion for 2 minutes.
3. Add beef and sauté for 5 minutes more. Turn to brown evenly. Remove from pan and keep hot.
4. Add remaining oil to pan and sauté mushrooms.
5. Add beef and onions to pan with seasonings.
6. Add yogurt and wine, and gently stir in. Heat, but do not boil.★
7. Serve with macaroni.

★ If thickening is desired, use 2 teaspoons of cornstarch. Calories are same as for flour, but cornstarch has double the thickening power. The calories for cornstarch are not included in the nutrients per serving given above. To add cornstarch, take small amount of wine and yogurt broth and put aside to cool. Stir in cornstarch. Add some of warm broth to cornstarch paste and stir. Then, add cornstarch mixture to pan.

Lean top round beef and plain low-fat yogurt transform this rich dish into a heart-healthy meal.

Black Skillet Beef With Greens and Red Potatoes

1 lb top round beef
1 Tbsp paprika
1½ tsp oregano
½ tsp chili powder
¼ tsp garlic powder
¼ tsp black pepper
⅛ tsp red pepper
⅛ tsp dry mustard
    as needed nonstick cooking spray
8 red-skinned potatoes, halved
3 cups onion, finely chopped
2 cups beef broth
2 cloves large garlic, minced
2 large carrots, peeled, cut into very thin, 2½-inch strips
2 bunch (½ lb) mustard greens, kale, or turnip greens, stems removed, coarsely torn

NUTRITIONAL FACTS	
CALORIES:	340
TOTAL FAT:	5 G
SATURATED FAT:	2 G
CHOLESTEROL:	64 MG
SODIUM:	109 MG
TOTAL FIBER:	8 G
PROTEIN:	30 G
CARBOHYDRATES:	45 G
POTASSIUM:	1,278 MG
YIELD:	6 SERVINGS
SERVING SIZE:	7 OZ

1. Partially freeze beef. Thinly slice across the grain into long strips ⅛ inch thick and 3 inches wide.
2. Combine paprika, oregano, chili powder, garlic powder, black pepper, red pepper, and dry mustard. Coat strips of meat with spice mixture.
3. Spray large, heavy skillet with nonstick coating. Preheat pan over high heat. Add meat and cook, stirring, for 5 minutes. Then add potatoes, onion, broth, and garlic, and cook covered over medium heat for 20 minutes. Stir in carrots, lay greens over top, and cook covered until carrots are tender, about 15 minutes.
4. Serve in large serving bowl with crusty bread for dunking.

Here's a one-dish meal that tastes even better than it sounds.

Quick Beef Casserole

½ lb lean ground beef

3½ cups tomatoes, diced

2 small carrots, diced

1 cup onion, chopped

1 cup celery, chopped

1 cup green pepper, cubed

1 cup frozen peas

1 cup uncooked rice

½ tsp black pepper

¼ tsp salt

¼ tsp paprika

NUTRITIONAL FACTS	
CALORIES:	201
TOTAL FAT:	5 G
SATURATED FAT:	2 G
CHOLESTEROL:	16 MG
SODIUM:	164 MG
TOTAL FIBER:	3 G
PROTEIN:	9 G
CARBOHYDRATES:	31 G
POTASSIUM:	449 MG
YIELD:	8 SERVINGS
SERVING SIZE:	1⅓ CUPS

1. In skillet, brown ground beef and drain off fat.
2. Add the rest of the ingredients. Mix well, adding 1½ cups of water. Cover and cook over medium heat until boiling. Reduce to low heat and simmer for 35 minutes. Serve hot.

Tired? Busy? You don't need hours to make healthy dishes. Try this one-skillet wonder.

Scrumptious Meat Loaf

1   lb ground beef, extra lean
2   cloves garlic, chopped
2   stalks scallion, chopped
1   cup tomatoes, fresh, blanched, chopped
½   cup (4 oz) tomato paste
¼   cup onion, chopped
¼   cup green peppers
¼   cup red peppers
¼   cup bread crumbs, finely grated
1   tsp orange rind, grated
½   tsp mustard, low-sodium
½   tsp hot pepper, chopped
½   tsp ground ginger
½   tsp thyme, crushed
¼   tsp ground black pepper
⅛   tsp ground nutmeg

NUTRITIONAL FACTS	
CALORIES:	193
TOTAL FAT:	9 G
SATURATED FAT:	3 G
CHOLESTEROL:	45 MG
SODIUM:	91 MG
TOTAL FIBER:	2 G
PROTEIN:	17 G
CARBOHYDRATES:	11 G
POTASSIUM:	513 MG
YIELD:	6 SERVINGS
SERVING SIZE:6,	1¼-INCH-THICK SLICES

1. Mix all ingredients together.
2. Place in 1-pound loaf pan (preferably with drip rack) and bake covered at 350° F for 50 minutes.
3. Uncover pan and continue baking for 12 minutes.

Got the meat loaf blahs? This recipe transforms the ordinary into the extraordinary.

Stir-Fried Beef and Potatoes

1½ lb sirloin steak
2 tsp vegetable oil
1 clove garlic, minced
1 tsp vinegar
⅛ tsp salt
⅛ tsp pepper
2 large onions, sliced
1 large tomato, sliced
3 cups boiled potatoes, diced

NUTRITIONAL FACTS	
CALORIES:	274
TOTAL FAT:	5 G
SATURATED FAT:	1 G
CHOLESTEROL:	56 MG
SODIUM:	96 MG
TOTAL FIBER:	3 G
PROTEIN:	24 G
CARBOHYDRATES:	33 G
POTASSIUM:	878 MG
YIELD:	6 SERVINGS
SERVING SIZE:	1¼ CUP

1. Trim fat from steak and cut into small, thin pieces.
2. In large skillet, heat oil and sauté garlic until golden.
3. Add steak, vinegar, salt, and pepper. Cook for 6 minutes, stirring beef until brown.
4. Add onion and tomato. Cook until onion is transparent. Serve with boiled potatoes.

Vinegar and garlic give this easy-to-fix dish its tasty zip.

Stir-Fried Beef and Chinese Vegetables

NUTRITIONAL FACTS	
CALORIES:	200
TOTAL FAT:	9 G
SATURATED FAT:	2 G
CHOLESTEROL:	40 MG
SODIUM:	201 MG
TOTAL FIBER:	3 G
PROTEIN:	17 G
CARBOHYDRATES:	12 G
POTASSIUM:	552 MG
YIELD:	6 SERVINGS
SERVING SIZE:	6 OZ

2 Tbsp dry red wine

1 Tbsp soy sauce

1½ tsp gingerroot, peeled, grated

½ tsp sugar

1 lb boneless round steak, fat trimmed, cut across grain into 1½-inch strips

2 Tbsp vegetable oil

2 medium onions, each cut into 8 wedges

½ lb fresh mushrooms, rinsed, trimmed, sliced

2 stalks (½ cup) celery, bias cut into ¼-inch slices

2 small green peppers, cut into thin lengthwise strips

1 cup water chestnuts, drained, sliced

2 Tbsp cornstarch

1. Prepare marinade by mixing together wine, soy sauce, ginger, and sugar.
2. Marinate meat in mixture while preparing vegetables.
3. Heat 1 Tbsp oil in large skillet or wok. Stir-fry onions and mushrooms for 3 minutes over medium–high heat.
4. Add celery and cook for 1 minute. Add remaining vegetables and cook for 2 minutes or until green pepper is tender but crisp. Transfer vegetables to warm bowl.
5. Add remaining 1 Tbsp oil to skillet. Stir-fry meat in oil for about 2 minutes, or until meat loses its pink color.
6. Blend cornstarch and ¼ cup of water. Stir into meat. Cook and stir until thickened. Then return vegetables to skillet. Stir gently and serve.

Stir-frying uses very little oil, as this dish shows.

Baked Pork Chops

6 lean center-cut pork chops,
 ½-inch thick★
1 egg white
1 cup evaporated skim milk
¾ cup cornflake crumbs
¼ cup fine dry bread crumbs
4 tsp paprika
2 tsp oregano
¾ tsp chili powder
½ tsp garlic powder
½ tsp black pepper
⅛ tsp cayenne pepper
⅛ tsp dry mustard
½ tsp salt
 as needed nonstick cooking spray

NUTRITIONAL FACTS	
CALORIES:	216
TOTAL FAT:	8 G
SATURATED FAT:	3 G
CHOLESTEROL:	62 MG
SODIUM:	346 MG
TOTAL FIBER:	1 G
PROTEIN:	25 G
CARBOHYDRATES:	10 G
POTASSIUM:	414
YIELD:	6 SERVINGS
SERVING SIZE:	1 CHOP

★ Try the recipe with skinless, boneless chicken or turkey parts, or fish—
bake for just 20 minutes.

1. Preheat oven to 375° F.
2. Trim fat from pork chops.
3. Beat egg white with evaporated skim milk. Place chops in milk mixture
and let stand for 5 minutes, turning once.
4. Meanwhile, mix cornflake crumbs, bread crumbs, spices, and salt.
5. Use nonstick cooking spray on 13- by 9-inch baking pan.
6. Remove chops from milk mixture and coat thoroughly with crumb
mixture.
7. Place chops in pan and bake at 375° F for 20 minutes. Turn chops and
bake for added 15 minutes or until no pink remains.

You can really sink your chops into these—they're made spicy and moist
with egg whites, evaporated milk, and a lively blend of herbs.

Shish Kabob

½ cup chicken broth
¼ cup red wine
1 lemon, juice only
2 Tbsp olive oil
1 tsp chopped garlic
¼ tsp salt
½ tsp rosemary
⅛ tsp black pepper
2 lb lean lamb, cut into 1-inch cubes
24 cherry tomatoes
24 mushrooms
24 pearl onions

NUTRITIONAL FACTS	
CALORIES:	274
TOTAL FAT:	12 G
SATURATED FAT:	3 G
CHOLESTEROL:	75 MG
SODIUM:	207 MG
TOTAL FIBER:	3 G
PROTEIN:	26 G
CARBOHYDRATES:	16 G
POTASSIUM:	728 MG
YIELD:	8 SERVINGS
SERVING SIZE:	1 KABOB, WITH 3 OZ OF MEAT

1. Combine oil, broth, wine, lemon juice, garlic, salt, rosemary, and pepper. Pour over lamb, tomatoes, mushrooms, and onions. Marinate in refrigerator for several hours or overnight.
2. Put together skewers of lamb, onions, mushrooms, and tomatoes. Broil 3 inches from heat for 15 minutes, turning every 5 minutes.

The delicious taste of these kabobs comes from the lively marinade of wine, lemon juice, rosemary, and garlic.

Spicy Veal Roast

1½ tsp cumin
½ tsp black pepper
½ tsp cinnamon
¼ tsp salt
3 lb boned lean veal shoulder, trimmed, rolled, tied
4 tsp olive oil
½ lb onions, peeled
½ clove garlic, peeled
2 tsp dried tarragon
4 sprigs fresh parsley
1 tsp thyme
1 bay leaf

NUTRITIONAL FACTS	
CALORIES:	206
TOTAL FAT:	8 G
SATURATED FAT:	3 G
CHOLESTEROL:	124 MG
SODIUM:	149 MG
TOTAL FIBER:	1 G
PROTEIN:	30 G
CARBOHYDRATES:	2 G
POTASSIUM:	459 MG
YIELD:	12 SERVINGS
SERVING SIZE:	3 OZ

1. Mix together cumin, pepper, cinnamon, and salt. Rub over roast.
2. Heat 2 teaspoons of oil in large skillet. Add onions, garlic, and tarragon. Cover and cook over low heat for 10 minutes. Set aside.
3. Heat remaining 2 teaspoons of oil in ovenproof pan large enough to hold all ingredients. Brown meat on all sides.
4. Add garlic-onion mixture. Add parsley, thyme, and bay leaf. Cover.
5. Bake in 325° F oven for 1½ hours, or until meat is tender.
6. Remove meat to serving platter. Skim fat from cooking juices. Remove bay leaf and parsley. Cut roast in ¼- to ½-inch slices. Pour a little cooking juice over roast and serve rest on side.

Skimming the fat from the cooking juices in this dish helps lower the fat content.

Chapter 10

♦ ♦ ❖ ♦ ♦ ❖ ♦ ♦ ❖ ♦ ♦ ❖ ♦ ♦ ❖ ♦ ♦ ❖ ♦ ♦

Poultry (Chicken and Turkey)

Your family and your heart will thank you for preparing the delicious dishes in this chapter. Poultry (chicken and turkey) is an extremely lean protein source and provides plenty of the vitamins B2, B6, B12, niacin, and pantothenic acid. These nutrients play many vital roles in our bodies. They assist in the formation of antibodies, allowing our bodies to fight disease. Without them, our cells would not be able to use fuel or oxygen, and hormones couldn't be produced. Iron and phosphorus are two main minerals prevalent in chicken and turkey. In addition to being involved in energy production, phosphorus fosters the growth of both bone and teeth. A deficiency in iron can result in the development of infections, anemia, and fatigue.

Fresh poultry is moist and has a subtle aroma. Avoid selecting poultry that has blemishes, discoloration, and bruises or shows signs of drying. Although dark chicken and turkey meat is still lean, it has almost double the calories and fat of white meat. Regardless of which choice you make, removing the skin will significantly reduce the fat content. Be careful when purchasing ground poultry though, it may have as much (or more) fat as ground beef because skin and dark meat are often used in this product. If you do decide to use ground poultry, make sure it is 100 percent ground chicken or turkey breast.

If you are not planning on preparing fresh poultry within two days of purchase, you should wrap over the original store packaging with air-tight plastic wrap and then freeze it. Whole poultry may be kept frozen for a year and poultry pieces for nine months. Bacteria grows rapidly on room temperature poultry so be sure to keep it cold. The back part of the refrigerator tends to be the coldest. It may take two to three days to defrost poultry in the refrigerator. If defrosting in the microwave is more convenient, use 50 percent power and cook the poultry immediately after defrosting.

Barbecued Chicken

3 lb chicken parts (breast, drumstick,
   and thigh), skin and fat removed
1 large onion, thinly sliced
1 cup chicken stock or broth, fat skimmed
   from top
3 Tbsp vinegar
3 Tbsp Worcestershire sauce
2 Tbsp brown sugar
1 Tbsp hot pepper flakes
1 Tbsp chili powder
   to taste black pepper

NUTRITIONAL FACTS	
CALORIES:	176
TOTAL FAT:	6 G
SATURATED FAT:	2 G
CHOLESTEROL:	68 MG
SODIUM:	240 MG
TOTAL FIBER:	1 G
PROTEIN:	24 G
CARBOHYDRATES:	7 G
POTASSIUM:	360 MG
YIELD:	8 SERVINGS
SERVING SIZE: 1 CHICKEN PART WITH SAUCE	

1. Place chicken in 13- by 9- by 2-inch pan.
   Arrange onions over top.
2. Mix together stock, vinegar, Worcestershire sauce, brown sugar, hot pepper flakes, chili powder, and pepper.
3. Pour mixture over chicken and bake at 350° F for 1 hour or until done.
   While cooking, baste occasionally.

Don't forget to remove the skin and fat to keep this zesty dish heart-
healthy.

Barbecued Chicken—Spicy Southern Style

2 cloves garlic, minced
5 Tbsp (3 oz) tomato paste
4 tsp white vinegar
2 tsp honey
1 tsp ketchup
1 tsp molasses
1 tsp Worcestershire sauce
¾ tsp cayenne pepper
¼ tsp onion powder
⅛ tsp black pepper
⅛ tsp ginger, grated
1½ lb chicken (breasts, drumsticks), skinless

NUTRITIONAL FACTS	
CALORIES:	176
TOTAL FAT:	4 G
SATURATED FAT:	LESS THAN 1 G
CHOLESTEROL:	81 MG
SODIUM:	199 MG
TOTAL FIBER:	1 G
PROTEIN:	27 G
CARBOHYDRATES:	7 G
POTASSIUM:	392 MG
YIELD:	6 SERVINGS
SERVING SIZE:	½ BREAST OR 2 SMALL DRUMSTICKS

1. Combine all ingredients except chicken in saucepan.
2. Simmer for 15 minutes.
3. Wash chicken and pat dry. Place it on large platter and brush with half of sauce mixture.
4. Cover with plastic wrap and marinate in refrigerator for 1 hour.
5. Place chicken on baking sheet lined with aluminum foil and broil for 10 minutes on each side to seal in juices.
6. Turn oven to 350° F and add remaining sauce to chicken. Cover chicken with aluminum foil and continue baking for 30 minutes.

Let yourself fall under the spell of this Southern-style, sweet, barbecue sauce.

Chicken Gumbo

1 tsp vegetable oil
¼ cup flour
3 cups low-sodium chicken broth
1½ lb chicken breast, skinless, boneless,
    cut into 1-inch strips
4 cloves garlic, finely minced
2 stalks scallion, chopped
1 cup (½ lb) white potatoes, cubed
1 cup onions, chopped
1 cup (½ lb) carrots, coarsely chopped
¼ cup celery, chopped
½ medium carrot, grated
2 tsp hot (or jalapeño) pepper
½ tsp thyme
½ tsp black pepper, ground
1 whole bay leaf
1 cup (½ lb) okra, sliced into ½-inch pieces

NUTRITIONAL FACTS	
CALORIES:	165
TOTAL FAT:	4 G
SATURATED FAT:	1 G
CHOLESTEROL:	51 MG
SODIUM:	81 MG
TOTAL FIBER:	2 G
PROTEIN:	21 G
CARBOHYDRATES:	11 G
POTASSIUM:	349 MG
YIELD:	8 SERVINGS
SERVING SIZE:	¾ CUP

1. Add oil to large pot and heat over medium flame.
2. Stir in flour. Cook, stirring constantly, until flour begins to turn golden brown.
3. Slowly stir in all broth using wire whisk. Cook for 2 minutes. Broth mixture should not be lumpy.
4. Add rest of ingredients except okra. Bring to boil, then reduce heat and let simmer for 20 to 30 minutes.
5. Add okra and let cook for 15 to 20 more minutes.
6. Remove bay leaf and serve hot in bowl or over rice.

Simple but filling—this dish feeds the need.

Chicken and Rice

6 chicken pieces (legs and breasts), skinless
2 tsp vegetable oil
2 tomatoes, chopped
1 medium carrot, grated
2 cloves garlic, chopped fine
½ cup onion, chopped
½ cup green pepper, chopped
¼ cup red pepper, chopped
¼ cup celery, diced
¼ cup corn, frozen
¼ cup fresh cilantro, chopped
⅛ tsp salt
⅛ tsp pepper
2 cups uncooked rice
½ cup frozen peas
2 oz Spanish olives
¼ cup raisins

NUTRITIONAL FACTS	
CALORIES:	448
TOTAL FAT:	7 G
SATURATED FAT:	2 G
CHOLESTEROL:	49 MG
SODIUM:	352 MG
TOTAL FIBER:	4 G
PROTEIN:	24 G
CARBOHYDRATES:	70 G
POTASSIUM:	551 MG
YIELD:	6 SERVINGS
SERVING SIZE:	1 CUP OF RICE AND 1 PIECE OF CHICKEN

1. In large pot, brown chicken pieces in oil.
2. Add 4 cups of water, tomatoes, green and red peppers, celery, carrots, corn, onion, cilantro, garlic, salt, and pepper. Cover and cook over medium heat for 20 to 30 minutes or until chicken is done.
3. Remove chicken from pot and place in refrigerator. Add rice, peas, and olives to pot. Cover pot and cook over low heat for about 20 minutes until rice is done.
4. Add chicken and raisins, and cook for another 8 minutes.

Let this Latino inspired dish—full of heart-healthy ingredients—inspire you.

Chicken and Spanish Rice

2 tsp vegetable oil
1 cup onions, chopped
¼ cup green peppers
1 can (8 oz) tomato sauce★
1¼ tsp garlic, minced
1 tsp parsley, chopped
½ tsp black pepper
5 cups cooked rice (in unsalted water)
3½ cups chicken breast, cooked, skin and
    bone removed, diced

NUTRITIONAL FACTS	
CALORIES:	406
TOTAL FAT:	6 G
SATURATED FAT:	2 G
CHOLESTEROL:	75 MG
SODIUM:	367 MG
TOTAL FIBER:	2 G
PROTEIN:	33 G
CARBOHYDRATES:	52 G
POTASSIUM:	527 MG
YIELD:	5 SERVINGS
SERVING SIZE:	1½ CUPS

★ Reduce sodium by using one 4-oz can of
"no salt added" tomato sauce and one 4-oz can of regular tomato
sauce. New sodium content for each serving is 226 mg.

1. In large skillet, sauté onions and green peppers in oil for 5 minutes on
medium heat.
2. Add tomato sauce and spices. Heat through.
3. Add cooked rice and chicken, and heat through.

This peppy dish is moderate in sodium but high in taste.

Chicken Marsala

¼ cup flour

¼ tsp salt

⅛ tsp black pepper

4 (5 oz total) chicken breasts, boned, skinless

1 Tbsp olive oil

½ cup Marsala wine

½ cup chicken stock, fat skimmed from top

½ cup mushrooms, sliced

½ lemon, juice only

1 Tbsp fresh parsley, chopped

NUTRITIONAL FACTS	
CALORIES:	285
TOTAL FAT:	8 G
SATURATED FAT:	2 G
CHOLESTEROL:	85 MG
SODIUM:	236 MG
TOTAL FIBER:	1 G
PROTEIN:	33 G
CARBOHYDRATES:	11 G
POTASSIUM:	348 MG
YIELD:	4 SERVINGS
SERVING SIZE: 1 CHICKEN BREAST WITH ⅓ CUP OF SAUCE	

1. Mix together flour, salt, and pepper. Coat chicken with seasoned flour.
2. In heavy-bottomed skillet, heat oil. Place chicken breasts in skillet and brown on both sides, then remove and set aside.
3. To skillet, add wine and stir until heated. Add stock, mushrooms, and lemon juice. Stir, reduce heat, and cook for about 10 minutes, until sauce is partially reduced.
4. Return browned chicken breasts to skillet. Spoon sauce over chicken.
5. Cover and cook for about 5 to 10 minutes or until chicken is done.
6. Serve sauce over chicken. Garnish with chopped parsley.

Want flavor without lots of salt and fat? Try this dish, which combines wine, lemon juice, and mushrooms into a delicious sauce.

Chicken Orientale

8 boneless, skinless chicken breasts, cut into
   chunks
   to taste black pepper
8 fresh mushrooms
8 whole white onions, parboiled
2 oranges, quartered
8 canned pineapple chunks, nonsweetened
8 cherry tomatoes
1 can (6 oz) frozen, concentrated apple
   juice, thawed
1 cup dry white wine
¼ cup vegetable oil
2 Tbsp soy sauce, low-sodium
2 Tbsp vinegar
   dash ginger, ground

NUTRITIONAL FACTS	
CALORIES:	359
TOTAL FAT:	11 G
SATURATED FAT:	2 G
CHOLESTEROL:	66 MG
SODIUM:	226 MG
TOTAL FIBER:	3 G
PROTEIN:	28 G
CARBOHYDRATES:	34 G
POTASSIUM:	756 MG
YIELD:	8 SERVINGS
SERVING SIZE:	½ KABOB

1. Sprinkle chicken breasts with pepper.
2. Thread 8 skewers as follows: chicken, mushroom, chicken, onion,
   chicken, orange quarter, chicken, pineapple chunk, cherry tomato.
   Place kabobs in shallow pan.
3. Combine remaining ingredients and spoon over kabobs. Marinate in
   refrigerator for at least 1 hour, then drain.
4. Broil kabobs 6 inches from heat for 15 minutes for each side. Brush
   with marinade every 5 minutes. After done, discard leftover marinade
   and serve kabobs.

Kabobs look as great as they taste, and these are made with no added salt
and very little oil, in order to keep them heart-healthy.

Chicken Ratatouille

1   Tbsp vegetable oil
4   medium chicken breast halves, skinned, fat removed, boned, and cut into 1-inch pieces
2   zucchini, about 7 inches long, unpeeled, thinly sliced
1   small eggplant, peeled, cut into 1-inch cubes
1   medium onion, thinly sliced
1   medium green pepper, cut into 1-inch pieces
½   lb fresh mushrooms, sliced
1   can (16 oz) whole tomatoes, cut up
1   clove garlic, minced
1   Tbsp fresh parsley, minced
1½ tsp dried basil, crushed
    to taste black pepper

NUTRITIONAL FACTS	
CALORIES:	266
TOTAL FAT:	8 G
SATURATED FAT:	2 G
CHOLESTEROL:	66 MG
SODIUM:	253 MG
TOTAL FIBER:	6 G
PROTEIN:	30 G
CARBOHYDRATES:	21 G
POTASSIUM:	1,148 MG
YIELD:	4 SERVINGS
SERVING SIZE:	1½ CUPS

1. Heat oil in large nonstick skillet. Add chicken and sauté for about 3 minutes or until lightly browned.
2. Add zucchini, eggplant, onion, green pepper, and mushrooms. Cook for about 15 minutes, stirring occasionally.
3. Add tomatoes, garlic, parsley, basil, and pepper. Stir and continue to cook for about 5 minutes or until chicken is tender.

It may be hard to say ratatouille, but this one-dish recipe will show you that it's very easy to eat.

Chicken Salad

3¼ cups chicken, cooked, cubed, skinless
¼ cup celery, chopped
3 Tbsp mayonnaise, low-fat
1 Tbsp lemon juice
½ tsp onion powder
⅛ tsp salt★

★ Reduce sodium by removing the ⅛ tsp of added salt. New sodium content for each serving is 127 mg.

NUTRITIONAL FACTS	
CALORIES:	183
TOTAL FAT:	7 G
SATURATED FAT:	2 G
CHOLESTEROL:	78 MG
SODIUM:	201 MG
TOTAL FIBER:	0 G
PROTEIN:	27 G
CARBOHYDRATES:	1 G
POTASSIUM:	240 MG
YIELD:	5 SERVINGS
SERVING SIZE:	¾ CUP

1. Bake chicken, cut into cubes, and refrigerate.
2. In large bowl, combine rest of ingredients, add chilled chicken and mix well.

Chill out with this simple, yet flavorful dish.

Chicken Stew

8 pieces chicken (breasts or legs)
3 medium tomatoes, chopped
2 cloves small garlic, minced
1 small onion, chopped
1½ tsp salt
1 tsp parsley, chopped
½ tsp pepper
¼ cup celery, finely chopped
2 medium potatoes, peeled, chopped
2 small carrots, chopped
2 bay leaves

NUTRITIONAL FACTS	
CALORIES:	206
TOTAL FAT:	6 G
SATURATED FAT:	2 G
CHOLESTEROL:	75 MG
SODIUM:	489 MG
TOTAL FIBER:	2 G
PROTEIN:	28 G
CARBOHYDRATES:	10 G
POTASSIUM:	493 MG
YIELD:	8 SERVINGS
SERVING SIZE: 1 PIECE OF CHICKEN	

1. Remove skin from chicken, along with any extra fat. In large skillet, combine chicken, 1 cup of water, tomatoes, garlic, onion, salt, parsley, and pepper. Tightly cover and cook over low heat for 25 minutes.
2. Add celery, potatoes, carrots, and bay leaves and continue to cook for 15 more minutes or until chicken and vegetables are tender. Remove bay leaves before serving.

This stew is as hearty as any, but healthier than most.

Crispy Oven-Fried Chicken

½ cup skim milk or buttermilk
1 tsp poultry seasoning
1 cup cornflakes, crumbled
1½ Tbsp onion powder
1½ Tbsp garlic powder
2 tsp black pepper
2 tsp dried hot pepper, crushed
1 tsp ginger, ground
8 pieces chicken, skinless (2 breasts, split, plus 4 drumsticks)
a few shakes of paprika

NUTRITIONAL FACTS

CALORIES:	249
TOTAL FAT:	4 G
SATURATED FAT:	1 G
CHOLESTEROL:	82 MG
SODIUM:	286 MG
TOTAL FIBER:	1 G
PROTEIN:	30 G
CARBOHYDRATES:	22 G
POTASSIUM:	339 MG

YIELD:	6 SERVINGS
SERVING SIZE:	½ BREAST OR
2 SMALL DRUMSTICKS	

1. Preheat oven to 350° F.
2. Add ½ teaspoon of poultry seasoning to milk.
3. Combine all other spices with cornflake crumbs and place in plastic bag.
4. Wash chicken and pat dry. Dip chicken into milk, shake to remove excess, then quickly shake in bag with seasoning and crumbs.
5. Refrigerate for 1 hour.
6. Remove from refrigerator and sprinkle lightly with paprika for color.
7. Evenly space chicken on greased baking pan.
8. Cover with aluminum foil and bake for 40 minutes. Remove foil and continue baking for an added 30 to 40 minutes or until meat can be easily pulled away from bone with fork. Drumsticks may require less baking time than breasts. (Do not turn chicken during baking.) Crumbs will form crispy "skin."

Kids will love this chicken—it tastes batter-dipped and fried, but is actually good for the heart.

Finger-Licking Curried Chicken

1 stalk scallion, chopped
8 cloves garlic, crushed
1 Tbsp hot pepper, chopped
1 Tbsp ginger, grated
1½ tsp curry powder
1 tsp thyme, crushed
1 tsp black pepper, ground
¾ tsp salt
½ tsp cayenne pepper, ground
1 Tbsp olive oil
8 pieces chicken, skinless (breast and drumsticks)
1 large onion, chopped
1 medium white potato, diced

NUTRITIONAL FACTS

CALORIES:	213
TOTAL FAT:	6 G
SATURATED FAT:	2 G
CHOLESTEROL:	81 MG
SODIUM:	363 MG
TOTAL FIBER:	1 G
PROTEIN:	28 G
CARBOHYDRATES:	10 G
POTASSIUM:	384 MG
YIELD:	6 SERVINGS
SERVING SIZE:	½ BREAST OR 2 SMALL DRUMSTICKS

1. Mix together scallion, garlic, hot pepper, ginger, curry powder, thyme, black pepper, salt, and cayenne pepper.
2. Sprinkle seasoning mixture on chicken.
3. Marinate for at least 2 hours in refrigerator.
4. Heat oil in skillet over medium flame. Add chicken and sauté.
5. Add water and allow chicken to cook over medium flame for 30 minutes.
6. Add onions and diced potatoes and cook for an added 45 minutes or until meat is tender.

The name tells all—ginger and curry powder make this dish irresistible.

Grilled Chicken With Green Chile Sauce

¼ cup olive oil
2 limes, juice only
½ tsp black pepper
¼ tsp oregano
4 chicken breasts, boneless, skinless
10 to 12 tomatillos, husks removed, cut in half
½ medium onion, quartered
2 cloves garlic, finely chopped
2 jalapeño peppers
2 Tbsp cilantro, chopped
¼ tsp salt
¼ cup low-fat sour cream

NUTRITIONAL FACTS	
CALORIES:	210
TOTAL FAT:	5 G
SATURATED FAT:	1 G
CHOLESTEROL:	73 MG
SODIUM:	91 MG
TOTAL FIBER:	3 G
PROTEIN:	29 G
CARBOHYDRATES:	14 G
POTASSIUM:	780 MG
YIELD:	4 SERVINGS
SERVING SIZE:	1 BREAST

1. Combine oil, juice from one lime, black pepper, and oregano in shallow, glass baking dish. Stir.
2. Place chicken breasts in baking dish and turn to coat each side. Cover dish and refrigerate overnight. Turn chicken periodically to marinate it on both sides.
3. Put ¼ cup of water, tomatillos, and onion into saucepan. Bring to gentle boil and cook uncovered for 10 minutes or until tomatillos are tender.
4. In blender, place cooked onion, tomatillos, and any remaining liquid. Add garlic, jalapeño peppers, cilantro, salt, and juice of second lime. Blend until all ingredients are smooth. Place sauce in bowl and refrigerate.
5. Place chicken breasts on hot grill and cook until done. Place chicken on serving platter. Spoon tablespoon of low-fat sour cream over each chicken breast. Pour sauce over sour cream.

In this recipe, the chicken is marinated to make it tender without using a lot of fat.

Jamaican Jerk Chicken

1 cup onion, pureed or finely chopped
6 cloves garlic, finely chopped
¼ cup vinegar
3 Tbsp brown sugar
1 Tbsp hot pepper, chopped
2 tsp oregano, crushed
2 tsp thyme, crushed
1½ tsp allspice, ground
1½ tsp black pepper, ground
1 tsp hot pepper, crushed, dried
½ tsp cinnamon, ground
½ tsp salt
8 pieces chicken, skinless (4 breasts,
    4 drumsticks)

NUTRITIONAL FACTS	
CALORIES:	199
TOTAL FAT:	4 G
SATURATED FAT:	1 G
CHOLESTEROL:	81 MG
SODIUM:	267 MG
TOTAL FIBER:	1 G
PROTEIN:	28 G
CARBOHYDRATES:	12 G
POTASSIUM:	338 MG
YIELDS:	6 SERVINGS
SERVING SIZE:	½ BREAST OR 2 SMALL DRUMSTICKS

1. Preheat oven to 350° F.
2. Combine all ingredients except chicken in large bowl. Rub seasoning mix over chicken and marinate in refrigerator for 6 hours or longer.
3. Evenly space chicken on nonstick or lightly greased baking pan.
4. Cover with aluminum foil and bake for 40 minutes. Remove foil and continue baking for an added 30 to 40 minutes or until the meat can be easily pulled away from the bone with a fork.

The spices and peppers in this dish will transport you to a whole new taste.

20-Minute Chicken Creole

4 medium chicken breast halves, skinless, boned, and cut into 1-inch strips★

1½ cups (1 large) green pepper, chopped

1½ cups celery, chopped

1 cup (14 oz) tomatoes, cut up★★

1 cup low-sodium chili sauce

¼ cup onion, chopped

2 cloves garlic, minced

1 Tbsp fresh basil (or 1 tsp dried)

1 Tbsp fresh parsley (or 1 tsp dried)

¼ tsp red pepper, crushed

¼ tsp salt

as needed nonstick cooking spray

NUTRITIONAL FACTS	
CALORIES:	274
TOTAL FAT:	5 G
SATURATED FAT:	1 G
CHOLESTEROL:	73 MG
SODIUM:	383 MG
TOTAL FIBER:	4 G
PROTEIN:	30 G
CARBOHYDRATES:	30 G
POTASSIUM:	944 MG
YIELD:	4 SERVINGS
SERVING SIZE:	1½ CUPS

★ For convenience, you can use uncooked boneless, skinless chicken breast.

★★ To cut back on sodium, try low-sodium canned tomatoes.

1. Spray deep skillet with nonstick cooking spray. Preheat pan over high heat.
2. Cook chicken in hot skillet, stirring, for 3 to 5 minutes or until no longer pink. Reduce heat.
3. Add green pepper, celery, tomatoes with juice, low-sodium chili sauce, onion, garlic, basil, parsley, crushed red pepper, and salt. Bring to boil and reduce heat. Simmer covered for 10 minutes.
4. Serve over hot cooked rice or whole wheat pasta.

This quick Southern dish contains no added fat and very little added salt in its spicy tomato sauce.

Very Lemony Chicken

1½ lb chicken breast, skinned, fat removed
½ cup fresh lemon juice
½ cup fresh lemon peel, sliced
1 medium onion, sliced
2 Tbsp white wine vinegar
1 Tbsp fresh oregano, chopped (or 1 tsp
   dried oregano, crushed)
½ tsp paprika
¼ tsp salt
   to taste black pepper

NUTRITIONAL FACTS	
CALORIES:	179
TOTAL FAT:	4 G
SATURATED FAT:	1 G
CHOLESTEROL:	73 MG
SODIUM:	222 MG
TOTAL FIBER:	2 G
PROTEIN:	28 G
CARBOHYDRATES:	8 G
POTASSIUM:	350 MG
YIELD:	4 SERVINGS
SERVING SIZE:	1 BREAST
WITH SAUCE	

1. Place chicken in 13- by 9- by 2-inch glass baking dish.
2. Mix lemon juice, lemon peel, onions, vinegar, and oregano. Pour over chicken, cover, and marinate in refrigerator several hours, turning occasionally, or overnight.
3. Sprinkle with paprika, salt, and pepper.
4. Cover and bake at 300° F for 30 minutes. Uncover and bake for added 30 minutes or until done.

This tangy chicken scores high on taste, while low in calories, saturated fat, and cholesterol.

Yosemite Chicken Stew and Dumplings

FOR STEW

  1 lb chicken, skinless, boneless, cut into 1-inch cubes
  ½ cup onion, coarsely chopped
  1 medium carrot, peeled, thinly sliced
  1 stalk celery, thinly sliced
  ¼ tsp salt
     to taste black pepper
  1 pinch ground cloves
  1 bay leaf
  1 tsp cornstarch
  1 package (10 oz) frozen peas
  1 tsp dried basil

FOR CORNMEAL DUMPLINGS

  1 cup yellow cornmeal
  ¾ cup sifted all-purpose flour
  2 tsp baking powder
  ½ tsp salt
  1 cup low-fat milk
  1 Tbsp vegetable oil

NUTRITIONAL FACTS	
CALORIES:	301
TOTAL FAT:	6 G
SATURATED FAT:	1 G
CHOLESTEROL:	43 MG
SODIUM:	471 MG
TOTAL FIBER:	5 G
PROTEIN:	24 G
CARBOHYDRATES:	37 G
POTASSIUM:	409 MG
YIELD:	6 SERVINGS
SERVING SIZE: 1¼ CUPS STEW WITH 2 DUMPLINGS	

TO PREPARE STEW:

1. Place chicken, onion, carrot, celery, salt, pepper, cloves, bay leaf, and 3 cups of water in large saucepan. Heat to boiling. Cover and reduce heat to simmer. Cook for about 30 minutes or until chicken is tender.

2. Remove chicken and vegetables from broth. Strain the broth.

3. Skim fat from the broth. Measure and, if necessary, add additional water to make 3 cups of liquid.

4. Add cornstarch to 1 cup of cooled broth and mix by shaking vigorously in jar with tight-fitting lid.

5. Pour mix into saucepan with remaining broth. Cook, stirring constantly, until liquid comes to boil and is thickened.

6. Add peas, basil, and reserved vegetables to sauce. Stir to combine.

7. Add chicken and heat slowly to boiling while preparing cornmeal dumplings.

TO PREPARE DUMPLINGS:

1. Put cornmeal, flour, baking powder, and salt into large mixing bowl.

2. Mix milk and oil. Add milk mixture all at once to dry ingredients. Stir just enough to moisten flour and evenly distribute liquid. Dough will be soft.

3. Drop by full tablespoons on top of stew. Cover saucepan tightly. Heat to boiling. Reduce heat to simmering, and steam for about 20 minutes. Do not lift cover.

This satisfying dish keeps the fat down so you can enjoy its dumplings without turning into one.

Autumn Turkey-Stuffed Cabbage

1 head cabbage
½ lb lean ground beef
½ lb ground turkey
2 small onions, one minced, one sliced
1 slice stale whole wheat bread, crumbled
⅛ tsp black pepper
1 can (16 oz) diced tomatoes
1 medium carrot, sliced
2 Tbsp brown sugar
1 Tbsp lemon juice
1 Tbsp cornstarch

NUTRITIONAL FACTS	
CALORIES:	235
TOTAL FAT:	9 G
SATURATED FAT:	3 G
CHOLESTEROL:	56 MG
SODIUM:	235 MG
TOTAL FIBER:	3 G
PROTEIN:	20 G
CARBOHYDRATES:	18 G
POTASSIUM:	545 MG
YIELD:	5 SERVINGS
SERVING SIZE:	2 ROLLS

1. Rinse and core cabbage. Carefully remove 10 outer leaves and place in saucepan. Cover with boiling water and simmer for 5 minutes. Remove cooked cabbage leaves and drain on paper towel.
2. Shred ½ cup of raw cabbage and set aside.
3. Brown ground beef, ground turkey, and minced onion in skillet. Drain fat.
4. Place cooked and drained meat mixture, bread crumbs, ¼ cup of water, and pepper in mixing bowl.
5. Drain tomatoes, reserving liquid, and add ½ cup tomato juice from can to meat mixture. Mix well. Place ¼ cup of filling on each parboiled, drained cabbage leaf. Fold. Place folded side down in skillet.
6. Add tomatoes, sliced onion, 1 cup of water, shredded cabbage, and carrot. Cover and simmer for about 1 hour or until cabbage is tender, basting occasionally.
7. Remove cabbage rolls to serving platter, keep warm.
8. Mix brown sugar, lemon juice, and cornstarch together in small bowl. Add to vegetables and liquid in skillet and cook, stirring occasionally, until thickened and clear. Serve over cabbage rolls.

This dish cuts the fat by mixing turkey and lean beef.

Spaghetti With Turkey Meat Sauce

1 lb ground turkey, lean
1 can (28 oz) tomatoes, cut up
1 cup green pepper, finely chopped
1 cup onion, finely chopped
2 cloves garlic, minced
1 tsp dried oregano, crushed
1 tsp black pepper
1 lb spaghetti, uncooked
   as needed nonstick cooking spray

NUTRITIONAL FACTS

CALORIES:	455
TOTAL FAT:	6 G
SATURATED FAT:	1 G
CHOLESTEROL:	51 MG
SODIUM:	248 MG
TOTAL FIBER:	5 G
PROTEIN:	28 G
CARBOHYDRATES:	71 G
POTASSIUM:	593 MG

YIELD:	6 SERVINGS
SERVING SIZE:	5 OZ OF SAUCE WITH 9 OZ OF COOKED SPAGHETTI

1. Coat large skillet with nonstick spray. Preheat over high heat.
2. Add turkey and cook, stirring occasionally, for 5 minutes. Drain and discard fat.
3. Stir in tomatoes with juice, green pepper, onion, garlic, oregano, and black pepper. Bring to boil. Reduce heat and simmer covered for 15 minutes, stirring occasionally. Remove cover and simmer for added 15 minutes. (For creamier sauce, give sauce a whirl in blender or food processor.)
4. Meanwhile, cook spaghetti in unsalted water. Drain well.
5. Serve sauce over spaghetti.

Turkey isn't just for Thanksgiving. Let it go Italian for this healthy, meaty spaghetti.

Turkey Meat Loaf

1 lb lean turkey, ground
½ cup regular oats, dry
¼ cup catsup
1 large egg
1 Tbsp onion, dehydrated

1. Combine all ingredients and mix well.
2. Bake in loaf pan at 350° F or to internal temperature of 165° F for 25 minutes.
3. Cut into five slices and serve.

Here's a healthier version of an old diner favorite.

NUTRITIONAL FACTS

CALORIES:	192
TOTAL FAT:	7 G
SATURATED FAT:	2 G
CHOLESTEROL:	103 MG
SODIUM:	214 MG
TOTAL FIBER:	1 G
PROTEIN:	21 G
CARBOHYDRATES:	23 G
POTASSIUM:	292 MG
YIELD:	5 SERVINGS
SERVING SIZE:	1 SLICE (3 OZ)

Chapter 11

◆ ◆ ❖ ◆ ◆ ❖ ◆ ◆ ❖ ◆ ◆ ❖ ◆ ◆ ❖ ◆ ◆ ❖ ◆ ◆

Fish

Omega-3 fatty acids are a type of fat that may lower your cholesterol. Some fish provide plenty of this nutrient. This is especially true with cold-water fish such as salmon and mackerel. Fish is loaded with protein and nearly void of saturated fat. Additionally, fish oils contain Vitamin A, which helps prevent night blindness, keeps body tissues healthy and allows for normal bone and teeth growth. Fish is also a source of vitamins B6, B12, niacin, and panthothenic acid— the benefits of which we've discussed before.

The most abundant minerals found in fish include phosphorus, iron, potassium, and iodine. Seafood is especially important when it comes to iodine. Along with table salt (which we discourage the use of), it is the best food source of this nutrient. Iodine helps form hormones that regulate the rate at which energy is used. An iodine deficiency can result in an enlarged thyroid and weight gain. Remember though, just because something is good doesn't mean more is better. Too much of a mineral can be toxic to the body.

Purchase whole fish with shiny, well-attached scales, firm flesh that springs back to touch, and bright, clear eyes. Also, the gills should be red or bright pink and the surface of the fish should be moist, bright, and lustrous. Avoid selecting fish with dry spots, discolorations or those with a strong fish smell. If fresh fish is not available, purchase fish that is still frozen rather than fish that has already been thawed.

It is preferable to prepare fresh fish within one day of purchase but if it's kept very cold, quality will remain for two days. Tightly wrap the fish in air-tight plastic and store it in the back of your refrigerator. Frozen fish can be stored for six months if it's lean and three months if it's of a fatter variety. Most fish are of the lean variety. Fatty fish rich in omega-3 fatty acids include: mackerel, spiny dogfish, herring, sardines, pilchards, bluefin tuna, lake trout, Atlantic sturgeon, salmon, and anchovies. Defrost frozen fish in the refrigerator and prepare it within one day of defrosting.

Baked Salmon Dijon

1 cup fat-free sour cream
3 Tbsp scallions, finely chopped
2 Tbsp Dijon mustard
2 Tbsp lemon juice
2 tsp dried dill
1½ lb salmon fillet with skin, cut in center
½ tsp garlic powder
½ tsp black pepper
  as needed fat-free cooking spray

NUTRITIONAL FACTS	
CALORIES:	196
TOTAL FAT:	7 G
SATURATED FAT:	2 G
CHOLESTEROL:	76 MG
SODIUM:	229 MG
TOTAL FIBER:	LESS THAN 1 G
PROTEIN:	27 G
CARBOHYDRATES:	5 G
POTASSIUM:	703 MG
YIELD:	6 SERVINGS
SERVING SIZE:	1 PIECE (4 OZ)

1. Whisk sour cream, scallions, mustard, lemon juice, and dill in small bowl to blend.
2. Preheat oven to 400° F. Lightly oil baking sheet with cooking spray.
3. Place salmon, skin side down, on prepared sheet. Sprinkle with garlic powder and pepper, then spread the sauce.
4. Bake salmon until just opaque in center, about 20 minutes.

This salmon entrée is easy to make and will be enjoyed by the whole family!

Baked Trout

2 lb trout fillet, cut into 6 pieces ★
1 medium tomato, chopped
½ medium onion, chopped
3 Tbsp lime juice (about 2 limes)
3 Tbsp cilantro, chopped
½ tsp olive oil
¼ tsp black pepper
¼ tsp salt
¼ tsp red pepper (optional)

★ Any kind of fish can be used.

NUTRITIONAL FACTS	
CALORIES:	236
TOTAL FAT:	9 G
SATURATED FAT:	3 G
CHOLESTEROL:	104 MG
SODIUM:	197 MG
TOTAL FIBER:	LESS THAN 1 G
PROTEIN:	34 G
CARBOHYDRATES:	2 G
POTASSIUM:	865 MG
YIELD:	6 SERVINGS
SERVING SIZE:	1 PIECE

1. Preheat oven to 350° F.
2. Rinse fish and pat dry. Place in baking dish.
3. In separate dish, mix remaining ingredients together and pour over fish.
4. Bake for 15 to 20 minutes or until fork-tender.

You'll reel them in with this nutritious delicious dish.

Catfish Stew and Rice

2 medium potatoes
1 can (14½ oz) tomatoes, cut up★
1 cup onion, chopped
1 cup (8 oz bottle) clam juice or water
2 cloves garlic, minced
½ head cabbage, coarsely chopped
1 lb catfish fillets
   as needed green onion, sliced
1½ Tbsp Chili and Spice Seasoning
   (see page 191)
2 cup cooked rice (white or brown)

NUTRITIONAL FACTS	
CALORIES:	363
TOTAL FAT:	8 G
SATURATED FAT:	2 G
CHOLESTEROL:	87 MG
SODIUM:	355 MG
TOTAL FIBER:	4 G
PROTEIN:	28 G
CARBOHYDRATES:	44 G
POTASSIUM:	1,079 MG
YIELD:	4 SERVINGS
SERVING SIZE: 1 CUP OF STEW WITH ½ CUP OF RICE	

★ Reduce the sodium by using low or no added sodium canned tomatoes.

1. Peel potatoes and cut into quarters.
2. In large pot, combine potatoes, tomatoes and their juice, onion, clam juice, 1 cup of water, and garlic. Bring to boil and reduce heat. Cook covered over medium-low heat for 10 minutes.
3. Add cabbage and return to boil. Reduce heat. Cook covered over medium-low heat for 5 minutes, stirring occasionally.
4. Meanwhile, cut fillets into 2-inch lengths. Coat with Chili and Spice Seasoning.
5. Add fish to vegetables. Reduce heat and simmer covered for 5 minutes or until fish flakes easily with fork.
6. Serve in soup plates. Garnish with sliced green onion, if desired. Serve with scoop of hot cooked rice.

Catfish isn't just Southern anymore. Everyone can go "down home" with this dish.

Fish Veronique

1 lb white fish (such as cod, sole, or turbot)
¼ tsp salt
⅛ tsp black pepper
¼ cup dry white wine
¼ cup chicken stock or broth, skim fat
  from top
1 Tbsp lemon juice
1 Tbsp soft margarine
2 Tbsp flour
¾ cup low-fat or skim milk
½ cup seedless grapes
  as needed nonstick cooking spray

NUTRITIONAL FACTS

CALORIES:	166
TOTAL FAT:	2 G
SATURATED FAT:	1 G
CHOLESTEROL:	61 MG
SODIUM:	343 MG
TOTAL FIBER:	LESS THAN 1 G
PROTEIN:	24 G
CARBOHYDRATES:	9 G
POTASSIUM:	453 MG

YIELD:	4 SERVINGS
SERVING SIZE: 1	FILLET WITH SAUCE

1. Spray 10- by 6-inch baking dish with non-stick spray. Place fish in pan and sprinkle with salt and pepper.
2. Mix wine, stock, and lemon juice in small bowl and pour over fish.
3. Cover and bake at 350° F for 15 minutes.
4. Melt margarine in small saucepan. Remove from heat and blend in flour. Gradually add milk and cook over moderately low heat, stirring constantly, until thickened.
5. Remove fish from oven, and pour liquid from baking dish into "cream" sauce, stirring until blended. Pour sauce over fish and sprinkle with grapes.
6. Broil about 4 inches from heat for 5 minutes or until sauce starts to brown.

Here's a trick to treat the taste buds: Remove the fat from the chicken broth and add low-fat milk to get a healthy sauce that tastes rich and looks creamy.

Mediterranean Baked Fish

2 tsp olive oil

1 large onion, sliced

1 can (16 oz) whole tomatoes, drained
   (reserve juice), coarsely chopped

1 cup dry white wine

½ cup tomato juice (reserved from canned
   tomatoes)

¼ cup lemon juice

¼ cup orange juice

1 clove garlic, minced

1 Tbsp fresh orange peel, grated

1 tsp fennel seeds, crushed

½ tsp dried oregano, crushed

½ tsp dried thyme, crushed

½ tsp dried basil, crushed

1 bay leaf

   to taste black pepper

1 lb fish fillets (sole, flounder, or sea perch)

NUTRITIONAL FACTS

CALORIES:	178
TOTAL FAT:	4 G
SATURATED FAT:	1 G
CHOLESTEROL:	56 MG
SODIUM:	260 MG
TOTAL FIBER:	3 G
PROTEIN:	22 G
CARBOHYDRATES:	12 G
POTASSIUM:	678 MG

YIELD: 4 SERVINGS

SERVING SIZE:4-OZ FILLET WITH SAUCE

1. Heat oil in large nonstick skillet. Add onion and sauté over moderate heat for 5 minutes or until soft.

2. Add all remaining ingredients except fish. Stir well and simmer uncovered for 30 minutes.

3. Arrange fish in 10- by 6-inch baking dish. Cover with sauce. Bake uncovered at 375° F for about 15 minutes or until fish flakes easily.

Taste the Mediterranean in this dish's tomato, onion, and garlic sauce.

Mouth-Watering Oven-Fried Fish

2 lb fish fillets

1 Tbsp lemon juice, fresh

¼ cup skim milk or 1% buttermilk

2 drops hot pepper sauce

1 tsp fresh garlic, minced

¼ tsp white pepper, ground

¼ tsp salt

¼ tsp onion powder

½ cup cornflakes, crumbled, or regular bread crumbs

1 Tbsp vegetable oil

1 fresh lemon, cut in wedges

NUTRITIONAL FACTS	
CALORIES:	183
TOTAL FAT:	2 G
SATURATED FAT:	LESS THAN 1 G
CHOLESTEROL:	80 MG
SODIUM:	325 MG
TOTAL FIBER:	1 G
PROTEIN:	30 G
CARBOHYDRATES:	10 G
POTASSIUM:	453 MG
YIELD:	6 SERVINGS
SERVING SIZE:	1 CUT PIECE

1. Preheat oven to 475° F.
2. Wipe fillets with lemon juice and pat dry.
3. Combine milk, hot pepper sauce, and garlic.
4. Combine pepper, salt, and onion powder with cornflake crumbs and place on plate.
5. Let fillets sit briefly in milk. Remove and coat fillets on both sides with seasoned crumbs. Let stand briefly until coating sticks to each side of fish.
6. Arrange on lightly oiled shallow baking dish.
7. Bake for 20 minutes on middle rack without turning.
8. Cut into 6 pieces. Serve with fresh lemon.

This heart-healthy dish can be made with many kinds of fish—to be enjoyed over and over.

Scallop Kabobs

3 medium green peppers, cut into
  1½-inch squares
1½ lb fresh bay scallops
1 pt cherry tomatoes
¼ cup dry white wine
¼ cup vegetable oil
3 Tbsp lemon juice
  dash garlic powder
  to taste black pepper
4 skewers

NUTRITIONAL FACTS	
CALORIES:	224
TOTAL FAT:	6 G
SATURATED FAT:	1 G
CHOLESTEROL:	43 MG
SODIUM:	355 MG
TOTAL FIBER:	3 G
PROTEIN:	30 G
CARBOHYDRATES:	13 G
POTASSIUM:	993 MG
YIELD:	4 SERVINGS
SERVING SIZE:	1 KABOB (6 OZ)

1. Parboil green peppers for 2 minutes.
2. Alternately thread green peppers, scallops, and cherry tomatoes on skewers.
3. Combine white wine, oil, lemon juice, garlic powder, and pepper.
4. Brush kabobs with wine mixture, then place on grill (or under broiler).
5. Grill for 15 minutes, turning and basting frequently.

These colorful kabobs use scallops, which are naturally low in saturated fat.

Spicy Baked Fish

1 lb cod (or other fish) fillet
1 Tbsp olive oil
1 tsp commercial spicy seasoning,
    salt free, or Hot 'N Spicy Seasoning mix
    (see recipe, page 140)
    as needed nonstick cooking spray

---

1. Preheat oven to 350° F. Spray casserole
    dish with nonstick cooking oil spray.
2. Wash and dry fish. Place in dish. Drizzle
    with oil and seasoning mixture.
3. Bake uncovered for 15 minutes or until fish
    flakes with fork. Cut into 4 pieces. Serve with rice.

This spicy seafood dish will delight everyone.

NUTRITIONAL FACTS

CALORIES:	134
TOTAL FAT:	5 G
SATURATED FAT:	1 G
CHOLESTEROL:	60 MG
SODIUM:	93 MG
TOTAL FIBER:	0 G
PROTEIN:	21 G
CARBOHYDRATES:	LESS THAN 1 G
POTASSIUM:	309 MG

YIELDS:	4 SERVINGS
SERVING SIZE:	1 PIECE (3 OZ)

Spinach-Stuffed Sole

  1 tsp olive oil
  ½ lb fresh mushrooms, sliced
  ½ lb fresh spinach, chopped
  1 clove garlic, minced
  ¼ tsp oregano leaves, crushed
1½ lb sole fillets or other white fish
  2 Tbsp sherry
  4 oz (1 cup) part-skim mozzarella cheese,
     grated
     as needed nonstick cooking spray

NUTRITIONAL FACTS	
CALORIES:	273
TOTAL FAT:	9 G
SATURATED FAT:	4 G
CHOLESTEROL:	95 MG
SODIUM:	163 MG
TOTAL FIBER:	2 G
PROTEIN:	39 G
CARBOHYDRATES:	6 G
POTASSIUM:	880 MG
YIELD:	4 SERVINGS
SERVING SIZE:	1 FILLET ROLL

1. Preheat oven to 400° F.
2. Coat 10- by 6-inch baking dish with nonstick cooking spray.
3. Heat oil in skillet and sauté mushrooms for about 3 minutes or until tender.
4. Add spinach and continue cooking for about 1 minute or until spinach is barely wilted. Remove from heat and drain liquid into prepared baking dish.
5. Add garlic and oregano to drained sautéed vegetables. Stir to mix ingredients.
6. Divide vegetable mixture evenly among fillets and place in center of each.
7. Roll each fillet around mixture and place seam-side down in prepared baking dish.
8. Sprinkle with sherry, then with grated mozzarella cheese. Bake for 15 to 20 minutes or until fish flakes easily. Lift out with slotted spoon.

Heart-healthy doesn't have to mean plain cooking, as this special dish shows.

Tuna Salad

2 can (6 oz each) tuna, water pack
½ cup raw celery, chopped
⅓ cup green onions, chopped
6½ Tbsp mayonnaise, reduced fat

---

1. Rinse and drain tuna for 5 minutes. Break apart with fork.
2. Add celery, onion, and mayonnaise, and mix well.

Perfect for a healthy lunchtime salad plate or sandwich.

NUTRITIONAL FACTS	
CALORIES:	146
TOTAL FAT:	7 G
SATURATED FAT:	1 G
CHOLESTEROL:	25 MG
SODIUM:	158 MG
TOTAL FIBER:	1 G
PROTEIN:	16 G
CARBOHYDRATES:	4 G
POTASSIUM:	201 MG
YIELD:	5 SERVINGS
SERVING SIZE:	½ CUP

Chapter 12

♦ ♦ ❖ ♦ ♦ ❖ ♦ ♦ ❖ ♦ ♦ ❖ ♦ ♦ ❖ ♦ ♦ ❖ ♦ ♦

Vegetables and Meatless Entrées

Meatless cookery has been around for years. Science has found that cultures consuming meatless cuisine, and thus less fat and calories, have fewer health related problems. Vegetables are nutrient dense— a great amount of nutrition is acquired by consuming small amounts. They are also filled with fiber which you now know is of enormous benefit. Vegetables contain a multitude of vitamins including B2, A, K, C, and folic acid. Vitamins are necessary for human survival, in fact, a lack of only one vitamin over time will result in death. Vitamin C, for example, repairs damaged tissues, promotes wound healing, increases resistance to infection and maintains healthy gums, bones and teeth. Inadequate consumption of folic acid may result in giving birth to a child with spina bifida or developing weakness, diarrhea, irritability, anemia, unintended weight loss, and a sore red tongue. Prevalent minerals in vegetables include calcium, copper, iron, manganese, and potassium. People consuming inadequate amounts of calcium have higher rates of high blood pressure, while eating potassium rich diets helps to protect others from developing the condition. Each vegetable varies in its specific vitamin and mineral content, so consuming three to five servings of a variety of vegetables each day is wise. The tasty recipes in this chapter will make meeting that goal a breeze.

Obviously, fresh vegetables offer the most when it comes to nutrition. Frozen vegetables take second place, but even canned vegetables are of nutritional value. The United States Department of Agriculture (USDA) has established grade standards for most fresh vegetables. Use of these standards is voluntary but most packers grade their vegetables and some even mark consumer packages with the grade. U.S. Grade A vegetables are of outstanding quality. They are tender, fresh, have good color and are essentially free from bruises and decay. Vegetables marked U.S. Grade B remain excellent in quality but their color and tenderness is not as good as those marked Grade A. U.S. Grade C vegetables are nutritious. They are, however, less uniform in both color and flavor and are more mature. Overall, the freshest vegetables are those that are crisp and are bright in color. As previously stated, most fresh vegetables can be stored for two to five days. Root vegetables can be stored longer—for a week or more.

Storing canned vegetables at a temperature below 75 degrees allows them to retain their quality for about a year. Avoid purchasing cans that are swollen at the ends or have dents which have pierced the metal or loosened the seam. To retain the quality of frozen vegetables, they should be stored as rapidly as possible. Frozen vegetables will keep for about two years if stored at an optimal freezer temperature range of 0 to 20 degrees.

Black Beans With Rice

1 lb black beans, dry
1½ cups onion, chopped
1 medium green pepper, coarsely chopped
1 clove garlic, minced
1 Tbsp vegetable oil
½ tsp salt
2 bay leaves
1 Tbsp vinegar (or lemon juice)
6 cups rice, cooked in unsalted water
1 jar (4 oz) sliced pimento, drained
1 lemon, cut into wedges

NUTRITIONAL FACTS	
CALORIES:	508
TOTAL FAT:	4 G
SATURATED FAT:	1 G
CHOLESTEROL:	0 MG
SODIUM:	206 MG
TOTAL FIBER:	14 G
PROTEIN:	21 G
CARBOHYDRATES:	98 G
POTASSIUM:	852 MG
YIELD:	6 SERVINGS
SERVING SIZE:	8 OZ

1. Pick through beans to remove bad ones.
   Soak beans overnight in cold water. Drain and rinse.
2. In large soup pot or Dutch oven, stir together beans, 7 cups of water, onion, green pepper, garlic, oil, salt, and bay leaves. Cover and boil for 1 hour.
3. Reduce heat and simmer, covered, for 3 to 4 hours or until beans are very tender. Stir occasionally, and add water if needed.
4. Remove and mash about a third of beans. Return to pot. Stir and heat through.
5. When ready to serve, remove bay leaves and stir in vinegar or lemon juice.
6. Serve over rice. Garnish with sliced pimento and lemon wedges.

A delicious Caribbean favorite that's made with very little added fat.

Caribbean Pink Beans

1 lb pink beans
2 medium plantains, finely chopped
1 large tomato, finely chopped
1 small red pepper, finely chopped
1 medium white onion, finely chopped
3 cloves garlic, finely chopped
1½ tsp salt

NUTRITIONAL FACTS	
CALORIES:	133
TOTAL FAT:	LESSTHAN 1 G
SATURATED FAT:	LESSTHAN 1 G
CHOLESTEROL:	0 MG
SODIUM:	205 MG
TOTAL FIBER:	5 G
PROTEIN:	6 G
CARBOHYDRATES:	28 G
POTASSIUM:	495 MG
YIELD:	16 SERVINGS
SERVING SIZE:	½ CUP

1. Rinse and pick through beans. Put beans in large pot and add 10 cups of water. Place pot in refrigerator and allow beans to soak overnight.
2. Cook beans until soft. Add more water, as needed, while beans are cooking.
3. Add plantains, tomato, pepper, onion, garlic, and salt. Continue cooking at low heat until plantains are soft.

This dish stays healthy by using beans prepared without lard or other fat. Try it with rice.

New Orleans Red Beans

1 lb dry red beans
1½ cups onion, chopped
1 cup celery, chopped
4 bay leaves
1 cup green peppers, chopped
3 Tbsp garlic, chopped
3 Tbsp parsley, chopped
2 tsp dried thyme, crushed
1 tsp salt
1 tsp black pepper

NUTRITIONAL FACTS	
CALORIES:	171
TOTAL FAT:	LESS THAN 1 G
SATURATED FAT:	LESS THAN 1 G
CHOLESTEROL:	0 MG
SODIUM:	285 MG
TOTAL FIBER:	7 G
PROTEIN:	10 G
CARBOHYDRATES:	32 G
POTASSIUM:	665 MG
YIELD:	8 SERVINGS
SERVING SIZE:	1¼ CUP

1. Pick through beans to remove bad ones. Rinse beans rinse thoroughly.
2. In large pot, combine beans, 2 quarts of water, onion, celery, and bay leaves. Bring to a boil. Reduce heat, cover, and cook over low heat for about 1½ hours or until beans are tender. Stir. Mash beans against side of pan.
3. Add green pepper, garlic, parsley, thyme, salt, and black pepper. Cook uncovered over low heat until creamy, about 30 minutes. Remove bay leaves.
4. Serve with hot cooked brown rice, if desired.

This vegetarian dish is virtually fat-free and entirely delicious.

Summer Vegetable Spaghetti

2 cups small yellow onions, cut in eighths

2 cups (about 1 lb) ripe tomatoes, peeled, chopped

2 cups (about 1 lb) yellow and green squash, thinly sliced

1½ cups (about ½ lb) fresh green beans, cut

2 Tbsp fresh parsley, minced

1 clove garlic, minced

½ tsp chili powder

¼ tsp salt

to taste black pepper

1 can (6 oz) tomato paste

1 lb spaghetti, uncooked

½ cup Parmesan cheese, grated

NUTRITIONAL FACTS

CALORIES:	271
TOTAL FAT:	3 G
SATURATED FAT:	1 G
CHOLESTEROL:	4 MG
SODIUM:	328 MG
TOTAL FIBER:	5 G
PROTEIN:	11 G
CARBOHYDRATES:	51 G
POTASSIUM:	436 MG

YIELD:	9 SERVINGS
SERVING SIZE:	1 CUP OF
SPAGHETTI AND ¾ CUP OF	
SAUCE WITH VEGETABLES	

1. Combine yellow onions, tomatoes, squash, green beans, parsley, garlic, chili powder, salt, pepper, and 2/3 cups of water in large saucepan. Cook for 10 minutes, then stir in tomato paste. Cover and cook gently for 15 minutes, stirring occasionally, until vegetables are tender.
2. Cook spaghetti in unsalted water according to package directions.
3. Spoon sauce over drained hot spaghetti. Sprinkle Parmesan cheese on top.

This lively vegetarian pasta dish is delicious hot or cold.

Vegetarian Spaghetti Sauce

2 Tbsp olive oil
3 cloves garlic, chopped
2 small onions, chopped
1¼ cup zucchini, sliced
1 can (8 oz) tomato sauce
1 can (6 oz) tomato paste★
2 medium tomatoes, chopped
1 Tbsp oregano, dried
1 Tbsp basil, dried

NUTRITIONAL FACTS	
CALORIES:	102
TOTAL FAT:	5 G
SATURATED FAT:	1 G
CHOLESTEROL:	0 MG
SODIUM:	459 MG
TOTAL FIBER:	5 G
PROTEIN:	3 G
CARBOHYDRATES:	14 G
POTASSIUM:	623 MG
YIELD:	6 SERVINGS
SERVING SIZE:	¾ CUP

★ Reduce sodium by using 6-oz can of "no salt added" tomato paste. New sodium content for each serving is 260 mg.

1. In medium skillet, heat oil. Sauté garlic, onions, and zucchini in oil for 5 minutes on medium heat.
2. Add remaining ingredients and 1 cup of water and simmer, covered, for 45 minutes. Serve over spaghetti.

Simple and simply delicious—here's a healthy sauce to serve with spaghetti or other pasta.

Zucchini Lasagna

¾ cup part-skim mozzarella cheese, grated

¼ cup Parmesan cheese, grated

1½ cup fat-free cottage cheese★

2½ cups no salt added tomato sauce

¼ cup onion, chopped

1 clove garlic

2 tsp basil, dried

2 tsp oregano, dried

⅛ tsp black pepper

½ lb lasagna noodles, cooked in unsalted
  water

1½ cups raw zucchini, sliced

NUTRITIONAL FACTS	
CALORIES:	276
TOTAL FAT:	5 G
SATURATED FAT:	2 G
CHOLESTEROL:	11 MG
SODIUM:	380 MG
TOTAL FIBER:	5 G
PROTEIN:	19 G
CARBOHYDRATES:	41 G
POTASSIUM:	561 MG
YIELD:	6 SERVINGS
SERVING SIZE:	1 PIECE

★ Use unsalted cottage cheese to reduce the sodium content. New sodium content for each serving is 196 mg.

1. Preheat oven to 350° F. Lightly spray 9- by 13-inch baking dish with vegetable oil spray.
2. In small bowl, combine ⅛ cup mozzarella and 1 Tbsp Parmesan cheese. Set aside.
3. In medium bowl, combine remaining mozzarella and Parmesan cheese with all of the cottage cheese. Mix well and set aside.
4. Combine tomato sauce with onion, garlic, basil, oregano, and pepper. Spread thin layer of tomato sauce in bottom of baking dish. Add a third of noodles in single layer. Spread half of cottage cheese mixture on top. Add layer of zucchini.
5. Repeat layering. Add thin coating of sauce. Top with noodles, sauce, and reserved cheese mixture. Cover with aluminum foil.
6. Bake for 30 to 40 minutes. Cool for 10 to 15 minutes. Cut into 6 portions.

Say, "Cheese," because this healthy version of a favorite comfort food will leave you smiling.

Fresh Cabbage and Tomato Salad

1   head small cabbage, sliced thinly
2   medium tomatoes, cut in cubes
1   cup radishes, sliced
2   Tbsp rice vinegar (or lemon juice)
2   Tbsp fresh cilantro, chopped
2   tsp olive oil
½   tsp black pepper
½   tsp red pepper
¼   tsp salt

NUTRITIONAL FACTS	
CALORIES:	43
TOTAL FAT:	1 G
SATURATED FAT:	LESSTHAN 1 G
CHOLESTEROL:	0 MG
SODIUM:	88 MG
TOTAL FIBER:	3 G
PROTEIN:	2 G
CARBOHYDRATES:	7 G
POTASSIUM:	331 MG
YIELD:	8 SERVINGS
SERVING SIZE:	1 CUP

1. In large bowl, mix together cabbage, tomatoes, and radishes.
2. In another bowl, mix together the rest of the ingredients and pour over vegetables.

Tempt your children to eat more vegetables with this refreshing, tasty salad.

Green Beans Sauté

1 lb fresh or frozen green beans, cut in
   1-inch pieces
1 Tbsp vegetable oil
1 large yellow onion, halved lengthwise,
   thinly sliced
½ tsp salt
⅛ tsp black pepper
1 Tbsp fresh parsley, minced

NUTRITIONAL FACTS	
CALORIES:	64
TOTAL FAT:	4 G
SATURATED FAT:	LESS THAN 1 G
CHOLESTEROL:	0 MG
SODIUM:	282 MG
TOTAL FIBER:	3 G
PROTEIN:	2 G
CARBOHYDRATES:	8 G
POTASSIUM:	161 MG
YIELD:	4 SERVINGS
SERVING SIZE:	¼ CUP

1. If using fresh green beans, cook in boiling water for 10 to 12 minutes or steam for 2 to 3 minutes until barely fork tender. Drain well. If using frozen green beans, thaw first.
2. Heat oil in large skillet. Sauté onion until golden.
3. Stir in green beans, salt, and pepper. Heat through.
4. Before serving, toss with parsley.

In this dish, green beans and onions are lightly sautéed in just 1 Tbsp of oil.

Italian Vegetable Bake

1   can (28 oz) tomatoes, whole

1   medium onion, sliced

½   lb fresh green beans, sliced

½   lb fresh okra, cut into ½-inch pieces
    (or ½ of 10-oz package frozen, cut)

¾   cup green pepper, finely chopped

2   Tbsp lemon juice

1   Tbsp fresh basil, chopped, or 1 tsp dried
    basil, crushed

1½ tsp fresh oregano leaves, chopped
    (or ½ tsp dried oregano, crushed)

3   medium (7-inch-long) zucchini, cut into
    1-inch cubes

1   medium eggplant, pared, cut into 1-inch cubes

2   Tbsp Parmesan cheese, grated

NUTRITIONAL FACTS	
CALORIES:	27
TOTAL FAT:	LESS THAN 1 G
SATURATED FAT:	LESS THAN 1 G
CHOLESTEROL:	1 MG
SODIUM:	86 MG
TOTAL FIBER:	2 G
PROTEIN:	2 G
CARBOHYDRATES:	5 G
POTASSIUM:	244 MG
YIELD:	18 SERVINGS
SERVING SIZE:	½ CUP

1. Drain and coarsely chop tomatoes. Save liquid. Mix together tomatoes, reserved liquid, onion, green beans, okra, green pepper, lemon juice, and herbs. Cover and bake at 325° F for 15 minutes.

2. Mix in zucchini and eggplant. Continue baking, covered, 60 to 70 minutes more or until vegetables are tender. Stir occasionally.

3. Just before serving, sprinkle top with Parmesan cheese.

Try this colorful, low-sodium baked dish, prepared without added fat.

Limas and Spinach

2 cup frozen lima beans
1 Tbsp vegetable oil
1 cup fennel, cut in 4-oz strips
½ cup onion, chopped
¼ cup low-sodium chicken broth
4 cups leaf spinach, washed thoroughly
1 Tbsp distilled vinegar
⅛ tsp black pepper
1 Tbsp raw chives

NUTRITIONAL FACTS	
CALORIES:	93
TOTAL FAT:	2 G
SATURATED FAT:	LESS THAN 1 G
CHOLESTEROL:	0 MG
SODIUM:	84 MG
TOTAL FIBER:	6 G
PROTEIN:	5 G
CARBOHYDRATES:	15 G
POTASSIUM:	452 MG
YIELD:	MAKES 7 SERVINGS
SERVING SIZE:	½ CUP

1. Steam or boil lima beans in unsalted water for about 10 minutes. Drain.
2. In skillet, sauté fennel and onions in oil.
3. Add beans and broth to onions and cover. Cook for 2 minutes.
4. Stir in spinach. Cover and cook until spinach has wilted, about 2 minutes.
5. Stir in vinegar and pepper. Cover and let stand for 30 seconds.
6. Sprinkle with chives and serve.

Your family will love vegetables cooked this way.

Smothered Greens

¼ lb smoked turkey breast, skinless
1 stalk scallion, chopped
¼ cup onion, chopped
2 cloves garlic, crushed
1 Tbsp fresh hot pepper, chopped
1 tsp ginger, ground
½ tsp thyme
¼ tsp cayenne pepper
¼ tsp cloves, ground
2 lb greens (mustard, turnip, collard, kale, or mixture)

NUTRITIONAL FACTS	
CALORIES:	80
TOTAL FAT:	2 G
SATURATED FAT:	LESS THAN 1 G
CHOLESTEROL:	16 MG
SODIUM:	378 MG
TOTAL FIBER:	4 G
PROTEIN:	9 G
CARBOHYDRATES:	9 G
POTASSIUM:	472 MG
YIELD:	5 SERVINGS
SERVING SIZE:	1 CUP

1. Place turkey, scallion, onion, garlic, hot pepper, ginger, thyme, cayenne pepper, cloves, and 3 cups of water into large saucepan and bring to boil.
2. Prepare greens by washing thoroughly and removing stems.
3. Tear or slice leaves into bite-size pieces.
4. Add greens to turkey stock. Cook for 20 to 30 minutes until tender.

These healthy greens get their rich flavor from smoked turkey, instead of fatback.

Vegetable Stew

1 cube vegetable bouillon, low-sodium
2 cups white potatoes, cut in 2-inch strips
2 cups carrots, sliced
4 cups summer squash, cut in 1-inch squares
1 can (15 oz) sweet corn, rinsed, drained
    (or 2 ears fresh corn, 1½ cup)
1 cup summer squash, cut in 4 chunks
1 cup onion, coarsely chopped
1 stalk scallion, chopped
2 cloves garlic, minced
½ small hot pepper, chopped
1 tsp thyme
1 cup tomatoes, diced (add other favorite vegetables, such as broccoli
    and cauliflower)

NUTRITIONAL FACTS	
CALORIES:	119
TOTAL FAT:	1 G
SATURATED FAT:	LESS THAN 1 G
CHOLESTEROL:	0 MG
SODIUM:	196 MG
TOTAL FIBER:	4 G
PROTEIN:	4 G
CARBOHYDRATES:	27 G
POTASSIUM:	524 MG
YIELD:	MAKES 8 SERVINGS
SERVING SIZE:	1¼ CUPS

1. Put 3 cups of water and bouillon in large pot and bring to a boil.
2. Add potatoes and carrots, and simmer for 5 minutes.
3. Add all summer squash, corn, onion, scallion, garlic, hot pepper, and thyme, and continue cooking for 15 minutes over medium heat.
4. Remove four chunks of squash and puree in blender.
5. Return pureed mixture to pot and let cook for 10 minutes more.
6. Add tomatoes and cook for another 5 minutes.
7. Remove from flame and let sit for 10 minutes to allow stew to thicken.

Here's a great new way to use summer vegetables.

Vegetables With a Touch of Lemon

½ head small cauliflower, cut into florets
2 cups broccoli, cut into florets
2 Tbsp lemon juice
1 Tbsp olive oil
1 clove garlic, minced
2 tsp fresh parsley, chopped

1. Steam broccoli and cauliflower until tender (about 10 minutes).
2. In small saucepan, mix the lemon juice, oil, and garlic, and cook over low heat for 2 or 3 minutes.
3. Put vegetables in serving dish. Pour lemon sauce over them. Garnish with parsley.

This heart-healthy sauce uses lemon juice and herbs for a tangy taste.

NUTRITIONAL FACTS

CALORIES:	22
TOTAL FAT:	2 G
SATURATED FAT:	LESSTHAN 1 G
CHOLESTEROL:	0 MG
SODIUM:	7 MG
TOTAL FIBER:	1 G
PROTEIN:	1 G
CARBOHYDRATES:	2 G
POTASSIUM:	49 MG
YIELD:	6 SERVINGS
SERVING SIZE:	½ CUP

Candied Yams

3 (1½ cups) medium yams
¼ cup brown sugar, packed
1 tsp flour, sifted
¼ tsp salt
¼ tsp ground cinnamon
¼ tsp ground nutmeg
¼ tsp grated orange peel
1 tsp soft tub margarine
½ cup orange juice

NUTRITIONAL FACTS	
CALORIES:	110
TOTAL FAT:	LESS THAN 1 G
SATURATED FAT:	LESS THAN 1 G
CHOLESTEROL:	0 MG
SODIUM:	115 MG
TOTAL FIBER:	2 G
PROTEIN:	1 G
CARBOHYDRATES:	25 G
POTASSIUM:	344 MG
YIELD:	6 SERVINGS
SERVING SIZE: ·	¼ CUP

1. Cut yams in half and boil until tender but firm (about 20 minutes). When cool enough to handle, peel and slice into ¼-inch pieces.
2. Combine sugar, flour, salt, cinnamon, nutmeg, and grated orange peel.
3. Place half of sliced yams in medium-size casserole dish. Sprinkle with spiced sugar mixture.
4. Dot with half the margarine.
5. Add second layer of yams, using the rest of the ingredients in the same order as above. Add orange juice.
6. Bake uncovered for 20 minutes in oven that was preheated to 350° F.

A bit of margarine and some orange juice make this dish taste lush and sweet.

Delicious Oven French Fries

4 (2 lb) large potatoes
1 tsp garlic powder
1 tsp onion powder
1 tsp white pepper
1 tsp hot pepper flakes
¼ tsp salt
¼ tsp allspice
1 Tbsp vegetable oil

NUTRITIONAL FACTS	
CALORIES:	238
TOTAL FAT:	4 G
SATURATED FAT:	1 G
CHOLESTEROL:	0 MG
SODIUM:	163 MG
TOTAL FIBER:	5 G
PROTEIN:	5 G
CARBOHYDRATES:	48 G
POTASSIUM:	796 MG
YIELD:	5 SERVINGS
SERVING SIZE:	1 CUP

1. Scrub potatoes and cut into ½-inch strips.
2. Place potato strips into 8 cups of ice water, cover, and chill for 1 hour or longer.
3. Remove potatoes and dry thoroughly.
4. Place garlic powder, onion powder, white pepper, pepper flakes, salt, and allspice in plastic bag.
5. Toss potatoes in spice mixture.
6. Brush potatoes with oil.
7. Place potatoes in nonstick shallow baking pan.
8. Cover with aluminum foil and place in 475° F oven for 15 minutes.
9. Remove foil and continue baking uncovered for additional 15 to 20 minutes or until golden brown. Turn fries occasionally to brown on all sides.

Find french fries hard to resist? Here's a version to give in to.

Garden Potato Salad

6 (about 3 lb) large potatoes, boiled in jackets, peeled, cut into 4–inch cubes
1 cup celery, chopped
½ cup green onion, sliced
2 Tbsp parsley, chopped
1 cup low-fat cottage cheese
¾ cup skim milk
3 Tbsp lemon juice
2 Tbsp cider vinegar
½ tsp celery seed
½ tsp dill weed
½ tsp dry mustard
½ tsp white pepper

NUTRITIONAL FACTS	
CALORIES:	145
TOTAL FAT:	1 G
SATURATED FAT:	LESS THAN 1 G
CHOLESTEROL:	2 MG
SODIUM:	122 MG
TOTAL FIBER:	3 G
PROTEIN:	6 G
CARBOHYDRATES:	29 G
POTASSIUM:	543 MG
YIELD:	10 SERVINGS
SERVING SIZE:	1 CUP

1. Place potatoes, celery, green onion, and parsley in a large bowl.
2. Meanwhile, in a blender or food processor, blend cottage cheese, milk, lemon juice, vinegar, celery seed, dill weed, dry mustard, and white pepper until smooth. Chill for 1 hour.
3. Pour chilled cottage cheese mixture over vegetables and mix well. Chill at least 30 minutes before serving.

Low-fat cottage cheese is the secret ingredient in this delicious dish.

Garlic Mashed Potatoes

2 (1 lb) large potatoes, peeled, quartered
2 cups skim milk
2 cloves garlic, large, chopped
½ tsp white pepper

NUTRITIONAL FACTS	
CALORIES:	142
TOTAL FAT:	LESS THAN 1 G
SATURATED FAT:	LESS THAN 1 G
CHOLESTEROL:	2 MG
SODIUM:	69 MG
TOTAL FIBER:	2 G
PROTEIN:	6 G
CARBOHYDRATES:	29 G
POTASSIUM:	577 MG
YIELD:	4 SERVINGS
SERVING SIZE:	¾ CUP

STOVETOP PREPARATION:

1. Cook potatoes, covered, in small amount of boiling water for 20 to 25 minutes or until tender. Remove from heat. Drain and recover.
2. Meanwhile, in small saucepan over low heat, cook garlic in milk until soft (about 30 minutes).
3. Add milk-garlic mixture and white pepper to potatoes. Beat with electric mixer on low speed, or mash with potato masher, until smooth.

MICROWAVE PREPARATION:

1. Scrub potatoes, pat dry, and prick with fork.
2. On plate, cook potatoes uncovered on 100 percent (high) power until tender (about 12 minutes), turning over once.
3. Let stand 5 minutes, then peel and quarter.
4. Meanwhile, in a 4–cup measuring glass, combine milk and garlic. Cook, uncovered, on 50 percent (medium) power until garlic is soft (about 4 minutes).
5. Continue to Step 3 of Stovetop Preparation.

Whether with saucepan or microwave, you can make this dish tasty without added fat or salt.

New Potato Salad

16 (5 cups) small new potatoes
¼ cup green onions, chopped
2 Tbsp olive oil
1 tsp dill weed, dried
¼ tsp black pepper

---

1. Thoroughly clean potatoes with vegetable brush and water.
2. Boil potatoes for 20 minutes or until tender.
3. Drain and cool potatoes for 20 minutes.
4. Cut potatoes into fourths and mix with onions, olive oil, dill, and pepper.
5. Refrigerate and serve.

Onions and spices give this very low-sodium dish plenty of zip.

NUTRITIONAL FACTS	
CALORIES:	187
TOTAL FAT:	6 G
SATURATED FAT:	1 G
CHOLESTEROL:	0 MG
SODIUM:	12 MG
TOTAL FIBER:	3 G
PROTEIN:	3 G
CARBOHYDRATES:	32 G
POTASSIUM:	547 MG
YIELD:	5 SERVINGS
SERVING SIZE:	1 CUP

Savory Potato Salad

6 (about 2 lb) medium potatoes

2 stalks celery, finely chopped

2 stalks scallion, finely chopped

¼ cup red bell pepper, coarsely chopped

¼ cup green bell pepper, coarsely chopped

1 Tbsp onion, finely chopped

1 egg, hard boiled, chopped

6 Tbsp light mayonnaise

1 tsp mustard

½ tsp salt

¼ tsp black pepper

¼ tsp dill weed, dried

NUTRITIONAL FACTS

CALORIES:	98
TOTAL FAT:	2 G
SATURATED FAT:	LESS THAN 1 G
CHOLESTEROL:	21 MG
SODIUM:	212 MG
TOTAL FIBER:	2 G
PROTEIN:	2 G
CARBOHYDRATES:	18 G
POTASSIUM:	291 MG
YIELD:	10 SERVINGS.
SERVING SIZE:	½ CUP

1. Wash potatoes, cut in half, and place in saucepan in cold water.

2. Cook covered over medium heat for 25 to 30 minutes or until tender.

3. Drain and dice potatoes when cool.

4. Add celery, scallion, bell peppers, onion, and egg to potatoes, and toss.

5. Blend together mayonnaise, mustard, salt, pepper, and dill weed.

6. Pour dressing over potato mixture, and stir gently to coat evenly.

7. Chill for at least 1 hour before serving.

Here's a potato salad that's both traditional and new—with a high taste-low-fat twist.

Wonderful Stuffed Potatoes

4   medium baking potatoes
¾   cup low-fat (1%) cottage cheese
¼   cup low-fat (1%) milk
2   Tbsp soft margarine
1   tsp dill weed
¾   tsp herb seasoning
4 to 6   drops hot pepper sauce
2   tsp Parmesan cheese, grated

NUTRITIONAL FACTS	
CALORIES:	113
TOTAL FAT:	3 G
SATURATED FAT:	1 G
CHOLESTEROL:	1 MG
SODIUM:	151 MG
TOTAL FIBER:	2 G
PROTEIN:	5 G
CARBOHYDRATES:	17 G
POTASSIUM:	293 MG
YIELD:	8 SERVINGS
SERVING SIZE:	½ POTATO

1. Prick potatoes with fork. Bake at 425° F for 60 minutes or until fork is easily inserted.

2. Cut potatoes in half lengthwise. Carefully scoop out potato, leaving about ½ inch of pulp inside shell. Mash pulp in large bowl.

3. By hand, mix in cottage cheese, milk, margarine, dill, herb seasoning, and hot pepper sauce. Spoon mixture into potato shells.

4. Sprinkle each top with ¼ teaspoon Parmesan cheese.

5. Place on baking sheet and return to oven. Bake for 15 to 20 minutes or until tops are golden brown.

Here's a lavish-tasting low-fat, low-cholesterol, low-sodium treat.

Chapter 13

◆ ◆ ✳ ◆ ◆ ✳ ◆ ◆ ✳ ◆ ◆ ✳ ◆ ◆ ✳ ◆ ◆ ✳ ◆ ◆

Grains (Pasta, Rice, and Bread)

Grains are actually seeds from a variety of grasses cultivated for food. Also called cereals, grains are low in fat and a great source of complex carbohydrates and fiber. They contain many vitamins including: vitamins D, E, B1, B2, B6, niacin, folic acid, biotin, and panthothenic acid. Grains are abundant in minerals as well. They are good sources of magnesium, chromium, manganese, molybdenum and selenium. Biotin helps the body produce energy and a deficiency in selenium could result in heart damage.

Grains have three parts—the bran, the germ, and the endosperm. The bran is the outer layer of the seed and contains the majority of vitamins, minerals and fiber found in the grain. Protein and some fat can be found in the germ. This is the part of the seed from which a new plant sprouts. The endosperm, also called the kernel, makes up the bulk of the seed and contains only small amounts of vitamins and minerals, it is, however, high in protein and carbohydrate. Refined grains are not as nutritious as whole grains because both the bran and germ have been removed. Whole grains have not had the bran extracted so they remain rich fiber sources and contain more vitamins and minerals.

When selecting grains look for the word whole on the package or listed in the ingredient list. To ensure quality and freshness, don't purchase grains that are past their "best if used by" date. Make sure you purchase them in sealed packages or airtight containers. Store them in these containers in a darkened area. This will protect them from air, moisture, and spoilage. Different grains have different storage times. Generally whole grains, such as brown rice, will keep for about six months and refined grains, such as white rice, will keep for nearly a year. You may also refrigerate or freeze grains to extend their storage time.

Chillin' Out Pasta Salad

2½ cups (8 oz) medium shell pasta
1 cup (8 oz) plain nonfat yogurt
2 Tbsp spicy brown mustard
2 Tbsp salt-free herb seasoning
1½ cup celery, chopped
1 cup green onion, sliced
1 lb small shrimp, cooked
3 cups (about 3 large) tomatoes, coarsely
  chopped

NUTRITIONAL FACTS	
CALORIES:	140
TOTAL FAT:	1 G
SATURATED FAT:	LESS THAN 1 G
CHOLESTEROL:	60 MG
SODIUM:	135 MG
TOTAL FIBER:	1 G
PROTEIN:	14 G
CARBOHYDRATES:	19 G
POTASSIUM:	295 MG
SERVINGS:	12
SERVING SIZE:	½ CUP

1. Cook pasta according to directions—but do not add salt to the water. Drain and cool.
2. In large bowl, stir together yogurt, mustard, and herb seasoning.
3. Add pasta, celery, and green onion, and mix well. Chill for at least 2 hours.
4. Just before serving, carefully stir in shrimp and tomatoes.

Cook up this taste feast and set the table for a new family favorite.

Classic Macaroni and Cheese

2 cups macaroni

½ cup onions, chopped

1¼ cup (4 oz) low-fat sharp cheddar cheese, finely shredded

½ cup evaporated skim milk

1 medium egg, beaten

¼ tsp black pepper

as needed nonstick cooking spray

NUTRITIONAL FACTS	
CALORIES:	200
TOTAL FAT:	4 G
SATURATED FAT:	2 G
CHOLESTEROL:	34 MG
SODIUM:	120 MG
TOTAL FIBER:	1 G
PROTEIN:	11 G
CARBOHYDRATES:	29 G
POTASSIUM:	119 MG
SERVINGS:	8
SERVING SIZE:	½ CUP

1. Cook macaroni according to directions—but do not add salt to the cooking water. Drain and set aside.
2. Spray casserole dish with nonstick cooking spray.
3. Preheat oven to 350° F.
4. Lightly spray saucepan with nonstick cooking spray. Add onions to saucepan and sauté for about 3 minutes.
5. In another bowl, combine macaroni, onions, cheese, milk, egg, pepper, and mix thoroughly.
6. Transfer mixture into casserole dish.
7. Bake for 25 minutes or until bubbly. Let stand for 10 minutes before serving.

This recipe proves you don't have to give up your favorite dishes to eat heart-healthy meals. Here's a low-fat version of a true classic.

Red Hot Fusilli

1 Tbsp olive oil
2 cloves garlic, minced
¼ cup fresh parsley, minced
4 cups ripe tomatoes, chopped
1 Tbsp fresh basil, chopped (or 1 tsp dried)
1 Tbsp oregano leaves, crushed
 (or 1 tsp dried)
¼ tsp salt
 to taste ground red pepper or cayenne
8 oz uncooked fusilli pasta (4 cup cooked)
½ lb (optional) cooked chicken breasts,
 diced into ½-inch pieces (¾ lb if raw)

---

1. Heat oil in medium saucepan. Sauté garlic and parsley until golden.
2. Add tomatoes, basil, oregano, salt, and red pepper. Cook uncovered over low heat for 15 minutes or until thickened, stirring frequently. If desired, add chicken and continue cooking for 15 minutes until chicken is heated through and sauce is thick.
3. Cook pasta in unsalted water until firm.
4. To serve, spoon sauce over pasta and sprinkle with coarsely chopped parsley. Serve hot as a main dish and cold for next day's lunch.

This lively dish is low in saturated fat and free of cholesterol.

NUTRITIONAL FACTS

EACH SERVING WITHOUT CHICKEN PROVIDES:	
CALORIES:	293
TOTAL FAT:	5 G
SATURATED FAT:	1 G
CHOLESTEROL:	0 MG
SODIUM:	168 MG
TOTAL FIBER:	4 G
PROTEIN:	9 G
CARBOHYDRATES:	54 G
POTASSIUM:	489 MG
EACH SERVING WITH CHICKEN PROVIDES:	
CALORIES:	391
TOTAL FAT:	8 G
SATURATED FAT:	1 G
CHOLESTEROL:	48 MG
SODIUM:	211 MG
TOTAL FIBER:	4 G
PROTEIN:	27 G
CARBOHYDRATES:	54 G
YIELD:	4 SERVINGS
SERVING SIZE:	1 CUP

Sweet and Sour Seashells

1 lb uncooked small seashell pasta
  (9 cup cooked)
2 Tbsp vegetable oil
¾ cup sugar
½ cup cider vinegar
½ cup wine vinegar
3 Tbsp prepared mustard
  to taste black pepper
1 jar (2 oz) sliced pimentos
2 small cucumbers
2 small onions, thinly sliced
18 leaves lettuce

NUTRITIONAL FACTS	
CALORIES:	158
TOTAL FAT:	2 G
SATURATED FAT:	LESS THAN 1 G
CHOLESTEROL:	0 MG
SODIUM:	35 MG
TOTAL FIBER:	2 G
PROTEIN:	4 G
CARBOHYDRATES:	31 G
POTASSIUM:	150 MG
YIELD:	18 SERVINGS
SERVING SIZE:	½ CUP

1. Cook pasta in unsalted water, drain, rinse with cold water, and drain again. Stir in oil.
2. Transfer to 4-quart bowl. In blender, place sugar, vinegars, ½ cup of water, prepared mustard, pepper, and pimento. Process at low speed for 15 to 20 seconds, or just enough so flecks of pimento can be seen. Pour over pasta.
3. Score cucumber peel with fork tines. Cut cucumber in half lengthwise, then slice thinly. Add to pasta with onion slices. Toss well.
4. Marinate, covered, in refrigerator for 24 hours. Stir occasionally.
5. Drain, and serve on lettuce. Drain the marinade before serving this dish in order to lower the fat and sodium—but keep all of the great taste.

Oriental Rice

1 cup chicken stock or broth, fat skimmed
  from top
1⅓ cups long grain white rice, uncooked
2 tsp vegetable oil
1 cup celery, finely chopped
2 Tbsp onion, finely chopped
½ cup pecans, chopped
½ cup water chestnuts, sliced
2 Tbsp green pepper, finely chopped
¼ tsp ground sage
¼ tsp nutmeg
  to taste black pepper

NUTRITIONAL FACTS	
CALORIES:	139
TOTAL FAT:	5 G
SATURATED FAT:	LESS THAN 1 G
CHOLESTEROL:	0 MG
SODIUM:	86 MG
TOTAL FIBER:	1 G
PROTEIN:	3 G
CARBOHYDRATES:	21 G
POTASSIUM:	124 MG
YIELD:	10 SERVINGS
SERVING SIZE:	½ CUP

1. Bring 1½ cups of water and stock to boil in medium-size saucepan.
2. Add rice and stir. Cover and simmer for 20 minutes.
3. Remove pan from heat. Let stand, covered, for 5 minutes or until all liquid is absorbed. Reserve.
4. Heat oil in large nonstick skillet.
5. Sauté celery and onion over moderate heat for 3 minutes. Stir in remaining ingredients, including reserved cooked rice. Fluff with fork before serving.

Skim off the fat from the chicken stock, use a minimum of oil, and don't add salt—and you'll create a dish that's flavorful and healthy.

Parmesan Rice and Pasta Pilaf

2 Tbsp olive oil
½ cup vermicelli, finely broken, uncooked
2 Tbsp onion, diced
1¼ cups chicken stock, hot
1 cup long grain white rice, uncooked
¼ tsp ground white pepper
1 bay leaf
2 Tbsp Parmesan cheese, grated

NUTRITIONAL FACTS	
CALORIES:	208
TOTAL FAT:	6 G
SATURATED FAT:	1 G
CHOLESTEROL:	2 MG
SODIUM:	140 MG
TOTAL FIBER:	1 G
PROTEIN:	5 G
CARBOHYDRATES:	33 G
POTASSIUM:	90 MG
YIELD:	6 SERVINGS
SERVING SIZE:	⅔ CUP

1. In large skillet, heat oil. Sauté vermicelli and onion until golden brown (about 2 to 4 minutes) over medium–high heat. Drain off oil.
2. Add stock, 1¼ cups of hot water, rice, pepper, and bay leaf. Cover and simmer for 15 to 20 minutes. Fluff with fork. Cover and let stand for 5 to 20 minutes. Remove bay leaf.
3. Sprinkle with cheese, and serve immediately.

Is it pilaf? Is it pasta? This dish is both—and healthy and tasty too.

Sunshine Rice

1½ Tbsp vegetable oil
1½ cups onion, finely chopped
1¼ cups celery, finely chopped, with leaves
½ cup orange juice
2 Tbsp lemon juice
  dash hot sauce
1 cup long grain white rice, uncooked
¼ cup slivered almonds

NUTRITIONAL FACTS	
CALORIES:	276
TOTAL FAT:	6 G
SATURATED FAT:	1 G
CHOLESTEROL:	0 MG
SODIUM:	52 MG
TOTAL FIBER:	5 G
PROTEIN:	7 G
CARBOHYDRATES:	50 G
POTASSIUM:	406 MG
YIELD:	4 SERVINGS
SERVING SIZE:	⅓ CUP

1. Heat oil in medium saucepan. Add onions and celery, and sauté until tender (about 10 minutes).
2. Add 1 cup of water, orange and lemon juices, and hot sauce. Bring to boil. Stir in rice and bring back to boil. Let stand covered until rice is tender and liquid is absorbed.
3. Stir in almonds. Serve immediately.

A citrus taste, combined with almonds, celery, and onions—but no added salt—make this side dish a new classic. Try it with fish.

Apricot-Orange Bread

1 package (6 oz) dried apricots, cut into small pieces

1 cup sugar

2 Tbsp margarine

1 egg, slightly beaten

1 Tbsp orange peel, freshly grated

3½ cups all-purpose flour, sifted

½ cup fat-free dry milk powder

2 tsp baking powder

1 tsp baking soda

1 tsp salt

½ cup orange juice

½ cup pecans, chopped

NUTRITIONAL FACTS	
CALORIES:	97
TOTAL FAT:	2 G
SATURATED FAT:	LESS THAN 1 G
CHOLESTEROL:	6 MG
SODIUM:	113 MG
TOTAL FIBER:	1 G
PROTEIN:	2 G
CARBOHYDRATES:	18 G
POTASSIUM:	110 MG
YIELD:	2 LOAVES
SERVING SIZE:	½-INCH SLICE

1. Preheat oven to 350° F. Lightly oil two, 9- by 5-inch loaf pans.
2. Cook apricots in 2 cups of water in covered medium-size saucepan for 10 to 15 minutes or until tender but not mushy. Drain and reserve ¾ cup liquid. Set apricots aside to cool.
3. Cream together sugar and margarine. By hand, beat in egg and orange peel.
4. Sift together flour, dry milk, baking powder, baking soda, and salt. Add to creamed mixture alternately with reserved apricot liquid and the orange juice.
5. Stir apricot pieces and pecans into batter.
6. Turn batter into prepared pans.
7. Bake for 40 to 45 minutes or until bread springs back when lightly touched in center.
8. Cool for 5 minutes in pans. Remove from pans and completely cool on wire rack before slicing.

This bread is low in all the right places—saturated fat, cholesterol, and sodium—without losing any taste and texture.

Banana-Nut Bread

1 cup ripe bananas, mashed
⅓ cup low-fat buttermilk
½ cup brown sugar, packed
¼ cup margarine
1 egg
2 cups all-purpose flour, sifted
1 tsp baking powder
½ tsp baking soda
½ tsp salt
½ cup pecans, chopped

NUTRITIONAL FACTS	
CALORIES:	133
TOTAL FAT:	5 G
SATURATED FAT:	1 G
CHOLESTEROL:	12 MG
SODIUM:	138 MG
TOTAL FIBER:	1 G
PROTEIN:	2 G
CARBOHYDRATES:	20 G
POTASSIUM:	114 MG
YIELD:	2 LOAVES
SERVING SIZE:	½-INCH SLICE

1. Preheat oven to 350° F. Lightly oil two, 9- by 5-inch loaf pans.
2. Stir together mashed bananas and buttermilk. Set aside.
3. Cream brown sugar and margarine together until light. Beat in egg. Add banana mixture and beat well.
4. Sift together flour, baking powder, baking soda, and salt. Add all at once to liquid ingredients. Stir until well blended.
5. Stir in nuts, and turn into prepared pans.
6. Bake for 50 to 55 minutes or until toothpick inserted in center comes out clean. Cool for 5 minutes in pans.
7. Remove from pans and complete cooling on a wire rack before slicing.

Bananas and low-fat buttermilk lower the fat for this old favorite, while keeping all the moistness.

Carrot-Raisin Bread

1½ cups all-purpose flour, sifted
½ cup sugar
1½ tsp ground cinnamon
 1 tsp baking powder
½ tsp salt
¼ tsp baking soda
¼ tsp ground allspice
 1 egg, beaten
 2 Tbsp vegetable oil
½ tsp vanilla
1½ cups carrots, finely shredded
¼ cup pecans, chopped
¼ cup golden raisins

NUTRITIONAL FACTS	
CALORIES:	99
TOTAL FAT:	3 G
SATURATED FAT:	LESS THAN 1 G
CHOLESTEROL:	12 MG
SODIUM:	97 MG
TOTAL FIBER:	1 G
PROTEIN:	2 G
CARBOHYDRATES:	17 G
POTASSIUM:	69 MG
YIELD:	2 LOAVES
SERVING SIZE:	½-INCH SLICE

1. Preheat oven to 350° F. Lightly oil two, 9- by 5-inch loaf pans.
2. Stir together flour, sugar, cinnamon, baking powder, salt, baking soda, and allspice in large mixing bowl. Make well in center of dry mixture.
3. In separate bowl, mix together ½ cup of water, egg, oil, vanilla, carrots, pecans, and raisins. Add mixture all at once to dry ingredients. Stir just enough to moisten and evenly distribute carrots.
4. Turn into prepared pan. Bake for 50 minutes or until toothpick inserted in center comes out clean.
5. Cool for 5 minutes in pan. Remove from pan and complete cooling on wire rack before slicing.

You don't need lots of oil and eggs to make a rich-tasting bread—as this recipe shows.

Good-for-You Cornbread

1 cup cornmeal

1 cup flour

¼ cup white sugar

1 tsp baking powder

1 cup 1% fat buttermilk

1 egg, whole

¼ cup tub margarine

1 tsp vegetable oil (to grease baking pan)

NUTRITIONAL FACTS

CALORIES:	178
TOTAL FAT:	6 G
SATURATED FAT:	1 G
CHOLESTEROL:	22 MG
SODIUM:	94 MG
TOTAL FIBER:	1 G
PROTEIN:	4 G
CARBOHYDRATES:	27 G
POTASSIUM:	132 MG
YIELD:	10 SERVINGS
SERVING SIZE:	1 SQUARE

1. Preheat oven to 350° F.
2. Mix together cornmeal, flour, sugar, and baking powder.
3. In another bowl, combine buttermilk and egg. Beat lightly.
4. Slowly add buttermilk and egg mixture to dry ingredients.
5. Add margarine, and mix by hand or with mixer for 1 minute.
6. Bake for 20 to 25 minutes in an 8- by 8-inch, greased baking dish. Cool. Cut into 10 squares.

This is not only good for you but also good in you—making it a healthy comfort food.

Homestyle Biscuits

2 cups flour
2 Tbsp sugar
2 tsp baking powder
¼ tsp baking soda
¼ tsp salt
⅔ cup 1% fat buttermilk
3⅓ Tbsp vegetable oil

NUTRITIONAL FACTS	
CALORIES:	99
TOTAL FAT:	3 G
SATURATED FAT:	LESS THAN 1 G
CHOLESTEROL:	LESS THAN 1 MG
SODIUM:	72 MG
TOTAL FIBER:	1 G
PROTEIN:	2 G
CARBOHYDRATES:	15 G
POTASSIUM:	102 MG
YIELD:	15 SERVINGS
SERVING SIZE:	1, 2-INCH BISCUIT

1. Preheat oven to 450° F.
2. In medium bowl, combine flour, sugar, baking powder, baking soda, and salt.
3. In small bowl, stir together buttermilk and all of the oil. Pour over flour mixture and stir until well mixed.
4. On lightly floured surface, knead dough gently for 10 to 12 strokes. Roll or pat dough to ¾-inch thickness. Cut with 2-inch biscuit or cookie cutter, dipping cutter in flour between cuts. Transfer biscuits to an ungreased baking sheet.
5. Bake for 12 minutes or until golden brown. Serve warm.

Update your homestyle biscuits with this easy low-fat recipe.

Chapter 14

◆ ◆ ❖ ◆ ◆ ❖ ◆ ◆ ❖ ◆ ◆ ❖ ◆ ◆ ❖ ◆ ◆ ❖ ◆ ◆

Desserts

Go ahead and indulge, the recipes included in this chapter are satisfying and delectable without containing too many calories or too much fat. In fact, more than half contain fewer than 200 calories and more than 90 percent provide a mere one gram of saturated fat or less. Additionally, they all have fiber, up to five grams per serving. So—you really can have your cake and eat it too!

Fruits are the key ingredients in many of these recipes. They provide a wealth of vitamins, including vitamins A and C. Minerals such as copper, phosphorus, potassium, and manganese, a component of enzymes needed for energy and protein metabolism, are abundant. As you know, fruits also provide fiber. Fruits that are in season and are grown by local farmers tend to be tastier and higher in quality than those shipped far distances. Visit your local farmer's market or produce stand if you can, and if not, ask the produce manager at your grocery store if any local fruits are available.

Apples, bananas, berries, and mangos are used most frequently in these recipes.

When choosing apples, look for those that are firm, crisp, and well colored. If the apple yields to slight pressure on the skin, it's overripe. Apples can be stored about a month in the refrigerator. Bananas generally keep three days at room temperature. Select firm, bright bananas free from bruises—bruised fruit will deteriorate fast. Also avoid bananas with a dull, grayish appearance because they won't ripen well. Pick berries that are colorful and firm. Stained or wet spots on non-plastic containers often indicate poor quality or spoilage. Leaky, moldy, mushy berries should also not be purchased. In the refrigerator, berries keep for two to three days. Ripe mangos have a fragrant aroma and are colored green and yellow with a little red mixed in. Those that are soft or bruised should not be bought. It is best to refrigerate mangos in a plastic bag away from vegetables. Their quality remains intact for three to five days.

Apple Coffee Cake

5 cups tart apples, cored, peeled, chopped

1 cup sugar

1 cup dark raisins

½ cup pecans, chopped

¼ cup vegetable oil

2 tsp vanilla

1 egg, beaten

2 cups all-purpose flour, sifted

2 tsp ground cinnamon

1 tsp baking soda

NUTRITIONAL FACTS	
CALORIES:	196
TOTAL FAT:	8 G
SATURATED FAT:	1 G
CHOLESTEROL:	11 MG
SODIUM:	67 MG
TOTAL FIBER:	2 G
PROTEIN:	3 G
CARBOHYDRATES:	31 G
POTASSIUM:	136 MG
YIELD:	20 SERVINGS
SERVING SIZE:	1, 3½-INCH BY 2½-INCH PIECE

1. Preheat oven to 350° F.
2. Lightly oil 13- by 9- by 2-inch pan.
3. In large mixing bowl, combine apples with sugar, raisins, and pecans. Mix well and let stand for 30 minutes.
4. Stir in oil, vanilla, and egg. Sift together flour, cinnamon, soda, and stir into apple mixture about a third at a time—just enough to moisten dry ingredients.
5. Turn batter into pan. Bake for 35 to 40 minutes. Cool cake slightly before serving.

Apples and raisins keep this cake moist—which means less oil and more health.

Banana Mousse

2 Tbsp low-fat milk
4 tsp sugar
1 tsp vanilla
1 medium banana, cut in quarters
1 cup plain low-fat yogurt
8 slices (¼ inch each) banana

NUTRITIONAL FACTS	
CALORIES:	94
TOTAL FAT:	1 G
SATURATED FAT:	1 G
CHOLESTEROL:	4 MG
SODIUM:	47 MG
TOTAL FIBER:	1 G
PROTEIN:	1 G
CARBOHYDRATES:	18 G
POTASSIUM:	297 MG
YIELD:	4 SERVINGS
SERVING SIZE:	½ CUP

1. Place milk, sugar, vanilla, and banana in blender. Process for 15 seconds at high speed until smooth.
2. Pour mixture into small bowl and fold in yogurt. Chill.
2. Spoon into four dessert dishes and garnish each with two banana slices just before serving.

This creamy dessert is a dream—yet low in saturated fat, cholesterol, and sodium.

Crunchy Pumpkin Pie

FOR CRUST

1 cup quick cooking oats
¼ cup whole wheat flour
¼ cup ground almonds
2 Tbsp brown sugar
¼ tsp salt
3 Tbsp vegetable oil
1 Tbsp water

FOR FILLING

¼ cup brown sugar, packed
½ tsp ground cinnamon
¼ tsp ground nutmeg
¼ tsp salt
1 egg, beaten
4 tsp vanilla
1 cup canned pumpkin
⅔ cup evaporated skim milk

NUTRITIONAL FACTS	
CALORIES:	169
TOTAL FAT:	7 G
SATURATED FAT:	1 G
CHOLESTEROL:	24 MG
SODIUM:	207 MG
TOTAL FIBER:	3 G
PROTEIN:	5 G
CARBOHYDRATES:	22 G
POTASSIUM:	223 MG
YIELD:	9 SERVINGS
SERVING SIZE:	⅑ OF 9-INCH PIE

TO PREPARE CRUST:

1. Preheat oven to 425° F.
2. Mix oats, flour, almonds, sugar, and salt in small mixing bowl.
3. Blend oil and water in measuring cup with fork or small wire whisk until blended.
4. Add oil mixture to dry ingredients and mix well. If needed, add small amount of water to hold mixture together.
5. Press into 9-inch pie pan, and bake for 8 to 10 minutes, or until light brown.
6. Turn down oven to 350° F.

TO PREPARE FILLING:

7. Mix sugar, cinnamon, nutmeg, and salt in bowl.
8. Add egg and vanilla, and mix to blend ingredients.
9. Add pumpkin and milk, and stir to combine.

continued on next page

PUTTING IT TOGETHER:

10. Pour filling into prepared pie shell.

11. Bake for 45 minutes at 350° F or until knife inserted near center comes out clean.

With only a small amount of oil in the crust and skim milk in the filling, this delicious pie is a heart-healthy treat.

Frosted Cake

FOR CAKE

2¼ cups cake flour

2¼ tsp baking powder

1¼ cups sugar

  4 Tbsp margarine

  4 eggs

  1 Tbsp orange peel

  1 tsp vanilla

¾ cup skim milk

FOR ICING

  3 oz low-fat cream cheese

  2 Tbsp skim milk

  6 Tbsp cocoa

  2 cups confectioners' sugar, sifted

½ tsp vanilla extract

NUTRITIONAL FACTS	
CALORIES:	241
TOTAL FAT:	5 G
SATURATED FAT:	2 G
CHOLESTEROL:	57 MG
SODIUM:	273 MG
TOTAL FIBER:	1 G
PROTEIN:	4 G
CARBOHYDRATES:	45 G
POTASSIUM:	95 MG
YIELD:	16 SERVINGS
SERVING SIZE:	1 SLICE

TO PREPARE CAKE:

1. Preheat oven to 325° F.

3. Grease 10-inch round pan (at least 2½ inches high) with small amount of cooking oil or use nonstick cooking oil spray. Powder pan with flour. Tap out excess flour.

4. Sift together flour and baking powder.

5. In separate bowl, beat together sugar and margarine until soft and creamy.

6. Beat in eggs, orange peel, and vanilla.

7. Gradually add flour mixture, alternating with milk, beginning and ending with flour.

8. Pour mixture into pan. Bake for 40 to 45 minutes or until done. Let cake cool for 5 to 10 minutes before removing from pan. Let cool completely before icing.

continued on next page

TO PREPARE ICING:

1. Cream together cream cheese and milk until smooth. Add cocoa. Blend well.

2. Slowly add sugar until icing is smooth. Mix in vanilla.

3. Smooth icing over top and sides of cooled cake.

Use skim milk and low-fat cream cheese—and you can bake your cake and eat it too.

Mango Shake

2 cups low-fat milk
4 Tbsp frozen mango juice (or 1 fresh
mango, pitted)
1 small banana
2 ice cubes

---

1. Put all ingredients into blender. Blend
until foamy. Serve immediately.

VARIATIONS
Instead of mango juice, try orange, papaya, or
strawberry juice.

Kids love this drink's creamy, sweet taste.

NUTRITIONAL FACTS

(WITH MANGO AND BANANA)

CALORIES:	106
TOTAL FAT:	2 G
SATURATED FAT:	1 G
CHOLESTEROL:	5 MG
SODIUM:	63 MG
TOTAL FIBER:	2 G
PROTEIN:	5 G
CARBOHYDRATES:	20 G
POTASSIUM:	361 MG

YIELD:	4 SERVINGS
SERVING SIZE:	¾ CUP

Mock-Southern Sweet Potato Pie

FOR CRUST

1¼ cups flour

¼ tsp sugar

⅓ cup skim milk

2 Tbsp vegetable oil

FOR FILLING

¼ cup white sugar

¼ cup brown sugar

½ tsp salt

¼ tsp nutmeg

3 large eggs, beaten

¼ cup canned evaporated skim milk

1 tsp vanilla extract

3 cups sweet potatoes, cooked, mashed

NUTRITIONAL FACTS	
CALORIES:	147
TOTAL FAT:	3 G
SATURATED FAT:	1 G
CHOLESTEROL:	40 MG
SODIUM:	98 MG
TOTAL FIBER:	2 G
PROTEIN:	4 G
CARBOHYDRATES:	27 G
POTASSIUM:	293 MG
YIELD:	16 SERVINGS
SERVING SIZE:	1 SLICE

TO PREPARE CRUST:

1. Preheat oven to 350° F.
2. Combine flour and sugar in bowl.
3. Add milk and oil to flour mixture.
4. Stir with fork until well mixed. Then form pastry into smooth ball with your hands.
5. Roll ball between two, 12-inch squares of waxed paper, using short, brisk strokes, until pastry reaches edge of paper.
6. Peel off top paper and invert crust into 9-inch pie plate.

TO PREPARE FILLING:

7. Combine sugars, salt, nutmeg, and eggs.
8. Add milk and vanilla. Stir.
9. Add sweet potatoes and mix well.

PUTTING IT TOGETHER:

10. Pour mixture into pie shell.

11. Bake for 60 minutes or until crust is golden brown. Cool and cut into 16 slices.

There's nothing fake about the flavor in this heart-healthy treat.

Old-Fashioned Bread Pudding With Apple-Raisin Sauce

FOR BREAD PUDDING

10 slices whole wheat bread
3 egg whites
1½ cups skim milk
¼ cup white sugar
2 tsp white sugar
¼ cup brown sugar
1 tsp vanilla extract
½ tsp cinnamon
¼ tsp nutmeg
¼ tsp clove
as needed vegetable oil spray

FOR APPLE-RAISIN SAUCE

1¼ cup apple juice
½ cup apple butter
½ cup raisins
2 Tbsp molasses
¼ tsp ground cinnamon
¼ tsp ground nutmeg
½ tsp orange zest (optional)

NUTRITIONAL FACTS

(WITH APPLE RAISIN SAUCE)

CALORIES:	233
TOTAL FAT:	3 G
SATURATED FAT:	1 G
CHOLESTEROL:	24 MG
SODIUM:	252 MG
TOTAL FIBER:	3 G
PROTEIN:	7 G
CARBOHYDRATES:	46 G
POTASSIUM:	390 MG

YIELD FOR BREAD PUDDING:	9 SERVINGS
YIELD FOR APPLE-RAISIN SAUCE:	2 CUPS
SERVING SIZE:	½ CUP

TO PREPARE BREAD PUDDING:

1. Preheat oven to 350° F.

2. Spray 8- by 8-inch baking dish with vegetable oil spray. Lay slices of bread in baking dish in two rows, overlapping like shingles.

3. In medium bowl, beat together egg whites, milk, ¼ cup white sugar, brown sugar, and vanilla. Pour egg mixture over bread.

4. In small bowl, stir together cinnamon, nutmeg, clove, and 2 teaspoons of white sugar.

5. Sprinkle spiced sugar mix over bread pudding. Bake pudding for 30 to 35 minutes, until it has browned on top and is firm to touch. Serve warm or at room temperature with warm apple-raisin sauce.

TO PREPARE APPLE-RAISIN SAUCE:

1. Stir all ingredients together in medium saucepan.

2. Bring to simmer over low heat. Let simmer for 5 minutes. Serve warm.

This old fashioned treat has been updated with a healthy spin. The sweet but healthy apple-raisin sauce makes a perfect topping—try it on fruit too.

1-2-3 Peach Cobbler

1 cup peach nectar

¼ cup pineapple juice or peach juice (if desired, use juice reserved from canned peaches)

2 Tbsp cornstarch

1 Tbsp vanilla extract

½ tsp ground cinnamon

2 can (16 oz each) peaches, packed in juice, drained, (or 1¾ lb fresh) sliced

1 Tbsp tub margarine

1 cup dry pancake mix

⅔ cup all–purpose flour

½ cup sugar

⅔ cup evaporated skim milk

 as needed nonstick cooking spray

1 Tbsp brown sugar

½ tsp nutmeg

NUTRITIONAL FACTS	
CALORIES:	271
TOTAL FAT:	4 G
SATURATED FAT:	LESS THAN 1 G
CHOLESTEROL:	LESS THAN 1 MG
SODIUM:	263 MG
TOTAL FIBER:	2 G
PROTEIN:	4 G
CARBOHYDRATES:	54 G
POTASSIUM:	284 MG
YIELD:	8 SERVINGS
SERVING SIZE:	1 PIECE

1. Combine peach nectar, pineapple or peach juice, cornstarch, vanilla, and cinnamon in saucepan over medium heat. Stir constantly until mixture thickens and bubbles.
2. Add sliced peaches to mixture.
3. Reduce heat and simmer for 5 to 10 minutes.
4. In another saucepan, melt margarine and set aside.
5. Lightly spray 8-inch-square glass dish with cooking spray. Pour hot peach mixture into dish.
6. In another bowl, combine pancake mix, flour, sugar, and melted margarine. Stir in milk. Quickly spoon this over peach mixture.
7. Combine brown sugar and nutmeg. Sprinkle on top of batter.
8. Bake at 400° F for 15 to 20 minutes or until golden brown.
9. Cool and cut into 8 pieces.

What could be better than peach cobbler straight from the oven? Try this healthier version of the classic favorite.

Rainbow Fruit Salad

FOR FRUIT SALAD

1 large mango, peeled, diced
2 cups fresh blueberries
2 cups fresh strawberries, halved
2 cups seedless grapes
2 bananas, sliced
2 nectarines, unpeeled, sliced
1 kiwi fruit, peeled, sliced

FOR HONEY–ORANGE SAUCE

⅓ cup unsweetened orange juice
2 Tbsp lemon juice
1½ Tbsp honey
¼ tsp ground ginger
  dash nutmeg

NUTRITIONAL FACTS	
CALORIES:	96
TOTAL FAT:	1 G
SATURATED FAT:	LESS THAN 1 G
CHOLESTEROL:	0 MG
SODIUM:	4 MG
TOTAL FIBER:	3 G
PROTEIN:	1 G
CARBOHYDRATES:	24 G
POTASSIUM:	302 MG
YIELD:	12 SERVINGS
SERVING SIZE:	4-OZ CUP

1. Prepare the fruit.
2. Combine all ingredients for sauce and mix.
3. Just before serving, pour honey–orange sauce over fruit.

You can't go wrong with this salad—it's juicy, fresh, naturally low in fat and sodium, and cholesterol free. Enjoy it as a salad or a dessert.

Rice Pudding

2 sticks cinnamon
1 cup rice
3 cups skim milk
⅔ cup sugar
½ tsp salt

---

1. Put 6 cups of water and cinnamon sticks into medium saucepan. Bring to boil.
2. Stir in rice. Cook on low heat for 30 minutes until rice is soft and water has evaporated.
3. Add skim milk, sugar, and salt. Cook for another 15 minutes until mixture thickens.

Skim milk gives a whole lot of flavor without whole milk's fat and calories.

NUTRITIONAL FACTS	
CALORIES:	372
TOTAL FAT:	1 G
SATURATED FAT:	LESS THAN 1 G
CHOLESTEROL:	3 MG
SODIUM:	366 MG
TOTAL FIBER:	1 G
PROTEIN:	10 G
CARBOHYDRATES:	81 G
POTASSIUM:	363 MG
YIELD:	5 SERVINGS
SERVING SIZE:	½ CUP

Summer Breezes Smoothie

1 cup fat-free, plain yogurt
1 cup pineapple, crushed, canned in juice
6 medium strawberries
1 medium banana
1 tsp vanilla extract
4 ice cubes

1. Place all ingredients in blender and puree until smooth.
2. Serve in frosted glass.

Here's a perfect low-fat thirst quencher.

NUTRITIONAL FACTS	
CALORIES:	121
TOTAL FAT:	LESS THAN 1 G
SATURATED FAT:	LESS THAN 1 G
CHOLESTEROL:	1 MG
SODIUM:	64 MG
TOTAL FIBER:	2 G
PROTEIN:	6 G
CARBOHYDRATES:	24 G
POTASSIUM:	483 MG
YIELD:	3 SERVINGS
SERVING SIZE:	1 CUP

Sweet Potato Custard

1   cup sweet potato, cooked, mashed
½   cup (about 2) small bananas, mashed
1   cup evaporated skim milk
2   egg yolks (or ⅓ cup egg substitute), beaten★
2   Tbsp brown sugar, packed
½   tsp salt
¼   cup raisins
1. Tbsp sugar
1   tsp ground cinnamon
    as needed nonstick cooking spray

NUTRITIONAL FACTS	
CALORIES:	160
TOTAL FAT:	2 G
SATURATED FAT:	1 G
CHOLESTEROL:	72 MG*
SODIUM:	255 MG
TOTAL FIBER:	2 G
PROTEIN:	5 G
CARBOHYDRATES:	32 G
POTASSIUM:	488 MG
YIELD:	6 SERVINGS
SERVING SIZE:	½ CUP

★ If using egg substitute, cholesterol will be lower.

1. In medium bowl, stir together sweet potato and banana.
2. Add milk, blending well.
3. Add egg yolks, brown sugar, and salt, mixing thoroughly.
4. Spray 1-quart casserole with nonstick cooking spray. Transfer sweet potato mixture to casserole dish.
5. Combine raisins, sugar, and cinnamon. Sprinkle over top of sweet potato mixture.
6. Bake in preheated 325° F oven for 40 to 45 minutes or until knife inserted near center comes out clean.

Sweet potatoes and bananas make this low-fat custard a dessert-lover's delight.

Tropical Fruit Compote

½ cup sugar

2 tsp fresh lemon juice

1 piece lemon peel

½ tsp rum or vanilla extract (optional)

1 pineapple, cored, peeled, cut into 8 slices

2 mangos, peeled, pitted, cut into 8 pieces

3 bananas, peeled, cut into 8 diagonal pieces
   to taste fresh mint leaves (optional)

NUTRITIONAL FACTS	
CALORIES:	148
TOTAL FAT:	LESS THAN 1 G
SATURATED FAT:	LESS THAN 1 G
CHOLESTEROL:	0 MG
SODIUM:	3 MG
TOTAL FIBER:	3 G
PROTEIN:	1 G
CARBOHYDRATES:	38 G
POTASSIUM:	310 MG
YIELD:	8 SERVINGS
SERVING SIZE:	1 CUP

1. In saucepan, combine ¾ cup of water with sugar, lemon juice, and lemon peel (and rum or vanilla extract, if desired). Bring to a boil, then reduce heat and add fruit. Cook at very low heat for 5 minutes.

2. Pour off syrup into cup.

3. Remove lemon rind from saucepan, and cool cooked fruit for 2 hours.

4. To serve, arrange fruit in serving dish.

Fresh or cooked, fruits are a great low calorie dessert. Top with low-fat or fat-free sour cream.

Winter Crisp

FOR FILLING

½ cup sugar

3 Tbsp all-purpose flour

1 tsp lemon peel, grated

5 cups apples, unpeeled, sliced

1 cup cranberries

¾ tsp lemon juice

FOR TOPPING

⅔ cup rolled oats

⅓ cup brown sugar, packed

¼ cup whole wheat flour

2 tsp ground cinnamon

1 Tbsp soft margarine, melted

NUTRITIONAL FACTS

(FOR WINTER CRISP)

CALORIES:	252
TOTAL FAT:	2 G
SATURATED FAT:	LESS THAN 1 G
CHOLESTEROL:	0 MG
SODIUM:	29 MG
TOTAL FIBER:	5 G
PROTEIN:	3 G
CARBOHYDRATES:	58 G
POTASSIUM:	221 MG

YIELD:	6 SERVINGS
SERVING SIZE:	1, ¾-INCH BY 2-INCH PIECE

1. Prepare filling by combining sugar, flour, and lemon peel in medium bowl. Mix well. Add lemon juice, apples, cranberries, and lemon juice. Stir to mix. Spoon into 6-cup baking dish.
2. Prepare topping by combining oats, brown sugar, flour, and cinnamon in small bowl. Add melted margarine. Stir to mix.
3. Sprinkle topping over filling. Bake in 375° F oven for approximately 40 to 50 minutes or until filling is bubbly and top is brown. Serve warm or at room temperature.

VARIATION–SUMMER CRISP

Prepare as directed above, but substitute 4 cups fresh or unsweetened frozen peaches and 3 cups fresh or unsweetened frozen blueberries for apples and cranberries. If using frozen fruit, thaw peaches completely (use without draining), but do not thaw blueberries before adding to mixture.

Only 1 Tbsp of margarine is used to make the crumb topping of this cholesterol-free, tart and tangy dessert.

Chapter 15

◆ ◆ ❖ ◆ ◆ ❖ ◆ ◆ ❖ ◆ ◆ ❖ ◆ ◆ ❖ ◆ ◆

Seasonings and Salad Dressings

Recipes found in this chapter require many herbs and spices. Although most call for dried herbs and spices, fresh can be used if you increase the amount specified by ⅔. Used properly, both herbs and spices can enhance flavor. If too much is used, it is likely the dish will be overpowered.

Choose fresh herbs that have a bright color, clean aroma and are free from browning or wilting. Fresh herbs will retain their quality for up to ten days if they are properly stored. Refrigerate herbs after submerging the stems in water, as you would cut flowers. Dried herbs should not be brown, rather they should have retained their original color. Smell dried spices prior to purchase to ensure they are aromatic and pungent. Dried spices will retain their quality up to six months if stored in airtight containers.

You will note that olive oil is an ingredient necessary for the preparation of our Vinaigrette Salad Dressing recipe. People are often confused about the different grades of olive oil. The difference is in how they are processed. Although they are processed differently, extra-virgin, virgin and regular olive oil are all excellent sources of monounsaturated fats that may reduce the risk of heart attack. As far as taste is concerned, extra-virgin olive oil has the most flavor and is best suited for salad dressing. The same can't be said for cooking because it tends to contain sediment and small particles of olives making it more likely to burn and smoke.

Chili and Spice Seasoning

¼ cup paprika

2 Tbsp dried oregano, crushed

2 tsp chili powder

1 tsp garlic powder

1 tsp black pepper

½ tsp red (cayenne) pepper

½ tsp dry mustard

Mix together all ingredients. Store in airtight container.

This spicy seasoning will heat up your catfish stew—and other dishes too.

NUTRITIONAL FACTS	
CALORIES:	26
TOTAL FAT:	1 G
SATURATED FAT:	0 G
CHOLESTEROL:	0 MG
SODIUM:	13 MG
TOTAL FIBER:	2 G
PROTEIN:	1 G
CARBOHYDRATES:	5 G
POTASSIUM:	180 MG
YIELD:	⅓ CUP
SERVING SIZE:	1 TBSP

Fresh Salsa

6 tomatoes, preferably Roma
  (or 3 large tomatoes)
½ medium onion, finely chopped
1 clove garlic, finely minced
½ avocado, diced (black skin)
2 jalapeño peppers, finely chopped
3 Tbsp cilantro, chopped
⅛ tsp oregano, finely crushed
⅛ tsp salt
⅛ tsp pepper
  to taste fresh lime juice

NUTRITIONAL FACTS	
CALORIES:	42
TOTAL FAT:	2 G
SATURATED FAT:	LESS THAN 1 G
CHOLESTEROL:	0 MG
SODIUM:	44 MG
TOTAL FIBER:	2 G
PROTEIN:	1 G
CARBOHYDRATES:	7 G
POTASSIUM :	337 MG
YIELD:	8 SERVINGS
SERVING SIZE:	½ CUP

1. Combine all ingredients in glass bowl.
2. Serve immediately or refrigerate and serve within 4 to 5 hours.

Fresh herbs add plenty of flavor to this salsa—so you use less salt.

Hot 'N Spicy Seasoning

1 Tbsp basil, dried
1½ tsp white pepper
1½ tsp thyme, dried
1¼ tsp garlic powder
1 tsp onion powder
½ tsp cayenne pepper
½ tsp black pepper

Mix all ingredients together. Store in an airtight container.

NUTRITIONAL FACTS	
CALORIES:	1
TOTAL FAT:	1 G
SATURATED FAT:	0 G
CHOLESTEROL:	0 MG
SODIUM:	0 MG
TOTAL FIBER:	0 G
PROTEIN:	0 G
CARBOHYDRATES:	LESS THAN 1 G
POTASSIUM:	4 MG
YIELD:	⅓ CUP
SERVING SIZE:	½ TEASPOON

Spices can make the ordinary extraordinary.
Here's a great all-purpose spice mix. Try this mix with meat, poultry, fish, or vegetable dishes. Use it instead of salt—even in the salt shaker.

Vinaigrette Salad Dressing

1 bulb garlic, separated into cloves, peeled
1 Tbsp red wine vinegar
1 Tbsp extra-virgin olive oil
½ tsp black pepper
¼ tsp honey

1. Place garlic cloves into small saucepan and pour in enough water (about ½ cup) to cover them.
2. Bring water to boil, then reduce heat and simmer until garlic is tender (about 15 minutes).
3. Reduce liquid to 2 Tbsp and increase heat for 3 minutes.
4. Pour contents into small sieve over bowl. With wooden spoon, mash garlic through sieve.
5. Whisk vinegar into garlic mixture, then mix in oil, pepper, and honey.

Try this recipe to dress up a salad for a special meal.

NUTRITIONAL FACTS	
CALORIES:	33
TOTAL FAT:	3 G
SATURATED FAT:	1 G
CHOLESTEROL:	0 MG
SODIUM:	0 MG
TOTAL FIBER:	0 G
PROTEIN:	0 G
CARBOHYDRATES:	1 G
POTASSIUM:	9 MG
YIELD:	4 SERVINGS
SERVING SIZE:	2 TBSP

Yogurt Salad Dressing

8 oz fat-free plain yogurt
¼ cup fat-free mayonnaise
2 Tbsp chives, dried
2 Tbsp dill, dried
2 Tbsp lemon juice

Mix all ingredients in bowl and refrigerate.

So easy—so healthy—so good. Try it!

NUTRITIONAL FACTS	
CALORIES:	23
TOTAL FAT:	0 G
SATURATED FAT:	0 G
CHOLESTEROL:	1 MG
TOTAL FIBER:	0 G
SODIUM:	84 MG
PROTEIN:	2 G
CARBOHYDRATES:	4 G
POTASSIUM:	104 MG
YIELD:	8 SERVINGS
SERVING SIZE:	2 TBSP

Glossary

◆ ◆ ❖ ◆ ◆ ❖ ◆ ◆ ❖ ◆ ◆ ❖ ◆ ◆ ❖ ◆ ◆ ❖ ◆ ◆

ATHEROSCLEROSIS: a type of artery disease characterized by patchy, nodular thickenings on the outer wall of the arteries.

BODY MASS INDEX: one of the most accurate ways to determine whether or not an adult is overweight, using weight and height to gauge body fat.

CHOLESTEROL: a waxy fat like substance in the blood. High levels contribute to heart disease.

HDL CHOLESTEROL: (high-density lipoprotein) a good blood cholesterol which helps to protect against heart disease.

HYDROGENATED FAT: polyunsaturated fats that have hydrogen added to them during food processing. These fats raise blood cholesterol.

HYPERTENSION: (high blood pressure) a condition that puts you at risk for heart disease, stroke and kidney disease. It is diagnosed when the force of blood against the walls of the arteries is too great, making your heart work harder than it should to pump blood throughout your body.

INSOLUBLE FIBER: (roughage) a component in plants that the body can't digest or absorb. It passes through the digestive tract largely intact and helps the colon function properly. This type of fiber also reduces cancer risk.

LDL CHOLESTEROL: (low-density lipoprotein) a bad blood cholesterol that increases the risk of heart disease.

MONOUNSATURATED FAT: a type of fat in the diet that helps to lower blood cholesterol.

OBESITY: a condition where one has too much body fat putting them at risk for health problems. Obesity is diagnosed if the BMI is equal to, or over 30.

OMEGA-3 FATTY ACIDS: a type of fat found is some species of fish that may reduce blood cholesterol levels.

PERCENT DAILY VALUE (%DV): is found on food labels. This tells you what percentage of your daily needs is being met for a particular nutrient per serving size specified. It is based on a 2,000 calorie per day "reference" diet.

PLANT STEROLS and STANOLS: naturally occurring substances found in plants and wood pulp similar in structure to cholesterol but not made by the human body. It is believed that they reduce the amount of cholesterol we absorb.

POLYUNSATURATED FAT: a type of dietary fat that is usually liquid at room temperature. This fat does not raise blood cholesterol.

SATURATED FAT: a type of dietary fat that is usually solid at room and refrigerator temperatures. This fat raises blood cholesterol.

SODIUM: a mineral that is a component of dietary salt and is involved in fluid regulation as well as nerve and muscle function. High intakes may lead to the development of high blood pressure.

SOLUBLE FIBER: (viscous) is a component in plants that the body can't digest or absorb. This type of fiber reduces the risk of heart disease and helps to control blood sugar levels.

TOTAL CHOLESTEROL: the sum of all types of cholesterol circulating through the blood.

TRANS FATTY ACID: a type of fat formed by manipulating the end of a fat molecule during food processing. Foods high in trans-fatty acids raise blood cholesterol.

Works Cited

◆ ❖ ◆ ❖ ◆ ❖ ◆ ❖ ◆ ❖ ◆ ❖ ◆ ❖ ◆ ❖ ◆

"Sample Diet Plans," pp 14, reproduced with permission from Martha McKittrick, R.D., C.D.E.

"Spotlight on the South Beach Diet," pp 16 (a review of Dr. Arthur Agatson's book), and "Low-Carb does not equal Low Calorie," pp 17, provided by Sari Budgazad, R.D., C.D.N.

"The Low-Carb Lingo," pp 18, provided by Sari Budgazad, R.D., C.D.N. Originally published in the University of California Berkeley Wellness Letter (January, 2004).

"Vitamin B12," pp 24, research provided by: www.mayoclinic.com. Heart Advisor Vol.2. No. 2. February 1999, pp 4-5.

"Trail Mix Ideas," pp 46–47, research provided by: Cleveland Clinic Heart Center www.clevelandclinic.org

"Heart Healthy Shopper," pp 66–70, Information adapted from:
Nancy Clark's "Sports Nutrition Guidebook," 1997,
Lyssie Lakatos R.D., L.D., C.D.N., C.P.T. and Tammy Lakatos Shames R.D., L.D., C.D.N., C.P.T.'s "Supermarket Savvy" (Powerpoint), and Brownell and Wadden's "Learn Program for Weight Control"

Recommended Dietary Allowances (RDA's) adapted from *Vitamins, Minerals and Dietary Supplements* by Marsha Hudnall (American Dietetic Association, 1998).

INDEX